4.95

Aromatherapy in Midwifery Practice

Aromatherapy in Midwifery Practice

Denise Tiran

SRN, SCM, ADM, MTD, PGCEA

Principal Lecturer, Complementary Therapies/
Midwifery Pathway Leader for the Diploma of Higher
Education in Complementary Therapy (Aromatherapy),
School of Health, University of Greenwich

 Baillière Tindall
LONDON PHILADELPHIA TORONTO SYDNEY TOKYO

Baillière Tindall   24–28 Oval Road
W. B. Saunders   London NW1 7DX

The Curtis Center
Independence Square West
Philadelphia, PA 19106–3399, USA

Harcourt Brace & Company
55 Horner Avenue
Toronto, Ontario, M8Z 4X6, Canada

Harcourt Brace & Company, Australia
30–52 Smidmore Street
Marrickville
NSW 2204, Australia

Harcourt Brace & Company, Japan
Ichibancho Central Building
22–1 Ichibancho
Chiyoda-ku, Tokyo 102, Japan

A catalogue record for this book is available from the British Library

ISBN 0–7020–1978–X

Typeset by J&L Composition Ltd, Filey, North Yorkshire
Printed and bound in Great Britain by WBC Book Manufacturers,
Bridgend, Mid Glamorgan

Contents

The colour plates are located between pages 152 and 153.

Acknowledgements

Fran Rawlings, School of Health, University of Greenwich, London, for reading the drafts and acting as mentor.

Dick Henson, School of Biological and Chemical Sciences, University of Greenwich, for advice on the chemistry of essential oils.

Students on the Diploma of Higher Education in Complementary Therapy (Aromatherapy) Pathway, University of Greenwich, for their encouragement.

Mothers and midwives at Queen Mary's Hospital, Sidcup, Kent, for their assistance—especially those who agreed to be photographed.

Sarah James, Publisher, Nursing and Midwifery, Baillière Tindall, and her Senior Editorial Assistant Karen Gilmour, for their unfailing support and enthusiam.

About this book

This book is not intended as a 'how to do it' manual, but rather provides a serious study of the values and dangers of aromatherapy in relation to pregnancy and childbearing. It is aimed at midwives who may be either novices or experts in using aromatherapy, but who wish to base their practice on currently available research findings. Managers considering (or being urged by staff to consider) the implementation of an aromatherapy service should find the factual information of help, as may lecturers preparing introductory sessions on complementary therapies for student midwives. Some of the issues raised may pose questions for debate, and the reference list will provide other sources of information to support that contained here.

Although the book is aimed primarily at midwives, general practitioners and obstetricians should find sections of interest to them. Aromatherapists who are not midwives can build on their existing knowledge so that they are able to treat pregnant clients safely.

The emphasis of the book is on balancing scientific knowledge with artistic skill; on weighing the pros and cons of safety with satisfaction; and on considering the practical issues pertinent to practice. Parts 1 and 2 are intended as cross-referencing guides, with the reader being able to 'dip in' to appropriate sections as required.

Aromatherapy should be something that is enjoyed, by both the recipient and the giver. Hopefully this book will facilitate midwives' confidence in administering a limited selection of essential oils to mothers, and to use the text as a reference for future practice. Good luck!

Chapter 1

Incorporation of Aromatherapy into Midwifery Practice

Aromatherapy is a science and an art in which essential oils derived from plants are used for their therapeutic properties. Essential oils can be administered via the skin through massage, in the bath or in a compress, via the mucous membranes in a douche or pessary, and via the respiratory tract through inhalation. Gastrointestinal administration is advocated in some cases, although this is generally used only by experienced clinical aromatherapists, who may also be qualified doctors.

Aromatherapy in Britain has, until recently, been more a part of the beauty therapy business, but it has long been recognized in Europe as having a part to play alongside conventional medical care. This has not been as an alternative but rather as a complement to medical treatment, sometimes called 'medecin douce' (gentle medicine), parallel medicine or, as Wells and Tschudin's (1994) book proclaims, a 'supportive' therapy.

Amongst the general public the popularity of aromatherapy has increased phenomenally in the past 15 years, with over 40 books on the subject in English alone, and the number of practising aromatherapists in the UK having risen from 100 to 5000. A 1991 survey by students from the Plymouth Business School asked 200 local people about their knowledge of aromatherapy (Tisserand, 1993). Over 70 per cent had heard of aromatherapy, 65 per cent wanted to learn more and 39 per cent had personally used essential oils. In 1992 approximately 2 per cent of all adults had purchased aromatherapy products, although most people did not immediately view aromatherapy as a form of medical treatment but rather as something that could de-stress them and make them feel good (Tisserand, 1993).

The popularity of aromatherapy and other manual therapies in the complementary medicine field, such as massage, reflexology and shiatsu, has risen even more rapidly in the past few years, markedly so amongst women. Aromatherapy has grown from a UK market size of £100,000 in 1981 to £20 million in 1991, and the number of training courses has risen from 5 to 80, but interest from men remains at a fairly constant low level of approximately 5 per cent. (Marsden, 1991). This may be due to the traditional perception of aromatherapy and massage as a luxury enjoyed by rich women, particularly when it involves the use of fragrances that have only recently begun to appeal to men. Marketing strategies for aromatherapy are not targeted towards men, so those who do advocate its use have generally 'discovered' it through female relatives and friends. The uninitiated view aromatherapy only as a means of relieving stress (also traditionally a woman's prerogative) and not until the last decade or so did aromatherapy's other benefits begin to be recognized by the general public and, latterly, by health professionals.

The move towards complementary therapies in health care

Aromatherapy is currently the fifth most popular 'alternative' therapy according to a survey of consumers published in the *Which?* report of 1992. The first four are osteopathy, chiropractic, acupuncture and homoeopathy, which can all be described as complete systems of medicine in their own right, so it is to the credit of aromatherapy that it ranks first of the truly 'supportive' therapies.

Aromatherapy is not alone amongst complementary therapies in gaining new converts; indeed almost one quarter of the British public has consulted an alternative practitioner at some time (British Medical Association, 1993). The British Medical Association has been forced to acknowledge that complementary medicine is no passing trend but is here to stay. Much of the acceptance and promotion of complementary therapies has come from nurses and midwives who are dissatisfied with the increase in technology in healthcare practice and who have observed the benefits of complementary therapies on their patients or clients. Many doctors are now following suit, particularly general practitioners who may employ complementary therapists in their surgeries if they consider it to be of value, for example in the relief of stress-related illnesses. Hospital consultants have, understandably, been somewhat slower to accept 'alternative' medicine, perhaps because they consider it a threat to their own autonomy or because patients referred to them require prompt treatment rather than that which may have fewer iatrogenic complications but which takes longer to be effective. They are also reluctant to condone other professionals administering to their patients substances of which they have little knowledge. It is ironic, however, that, on the one hand, some doctors dismiss the effects of aromatherapy as 'all in the mind' yet, on the other, express concern about possible interactions with prescribed medicines. In fact, the latter issue is far more pertinent but should not be a barrier to facilitating the use of essential oils that are considered safe for a particular client group. Many junior doctors are keen to learn more about the alternatives and recognize that a partnership needs to be developed between conventional and complementary practitioners; some medical schools now include an introduction to the subject in their undergraduate curricula.

Several health authorities are prepared to purchase complementary therapy services to improve care for their consumers, although others are reluctant to do so until more scientific evidence is available regarding efficacy and safety. At present, health authorities and trusts that are considering 'buying in' complementary medicine appear to prefer systems such as acupuncture, osteopathy, homeopathy and hypnotherapy, perhaps because these are often practised by doctors (commonly general practitioners) alongside their conventional treatment, whereas aromatherapy has a lower priority and is seen as useful only for conditions such as insomnia and anxiety (NAHAT, 1993).

One health authority has taken the step of actually employing a district clinical aromatologist; another has a complementary therapy MacMillan nurse; others 'allow' aromatherapists to offer their services on a voluntary basis. Where aromatherapy is available to National Health Service patients and clients in other areas, it is usually as a result of nurse- or midwife-led initiatives (Mack, 1995, p. 279) and is incorporated into their normal workload. Practitioners in certain clinical specialties, such as oncology, learning disabilities, midwifery and community care, are more enthusiastic about implementing aromatherapy services than those involved in acute care, although not exclusively so.

Within midwifery, requests from the women to use aromatherapy are sporadic, although occasionally a mother wishes to use essential oils for labour or may enquire about suitable oils to use in pregnancy. Midwives, however, are coming to view aromatherapy and other complementary therapies as additional strategies for symptom relief of, primarily, physiological disorders. They are keen to be able to return to the nurturing that staff shortages, heavy workloads and the increased technology of the past 10–15 years have denied mothers.

Evaluation and audit of maternity care is encouraging midwives to question the necessity of many traditional practices and to adapt care accordingly. The introduction of complementary therapies is just one means of enhancing care by offering women choice; part of what aromatherapy has to offer is a positive, individualized, woman-centred attitude in keeping with the philosophy of 'Changing Childbirth' (Department of Health, 1993). It could be argued that, where such an attitude exists within a maternity unit, aromatherapy will be only one way of providing a service which is satisfying for both mothers and midwives, and that other initiatives are likely to be in force, such as team midwifery, bereavement counselling services and water birth facilities. If this is the case, it is also probable that enthusiastic midwives will have managerial support and, hopefully, a good working relationship with the medical staff, so that the implementation of new initiatives can be worked through, without initial concerns or conflicts adversely affecting care of the mothers.

Historical perspectives

It is known that plants and their essences have been used for thousands of years, both for perfume and for therapeutic reasons. The term 'aromatherapie' was not used until the early twentieth century when Gattefosse began his experiments with the medicinal uses of essential oils, after burning his hand and discovering that lavender oil acted as an analgesic, antibacterial and wound-healing agent.

In ancient Egypt, embalming and mummification of the dead was achieved with essential oils, which were found to preserve, disinfect and deodorize the bodies, and Cleopatra is thought to have seduced Mark Antony with her lavish use of perfumes. The ancient Greeks also applied aromatic oils to their bodies as perfumes and medicines, and spread them around places of worship as incense. Medicinal use of plants in India dates back over 5000 years and is still the basis of Ayurvedic medicine today. There are many accounts of Roman centurions benefiting from the therapeutic properties of plants, for example chewing fennel seeds to suppress hunger as they marched to battle. The Bible also has several references to aromatic oils that were used to anoint or massage the feet—Mary Magdalen anointed Jesus with spikenard ointment before the Last Supper.

Knowledge gained from the Egyptians and Indians by the Greeks, especially around the time of Hippocrates over 400 years BC, was recorded as a means of passing information to future generations and at about AD 100 the Roman Dioscorides compiled a materia medica with details of several hundred plants. During the same period the Persian Ibn Sina, known to us as Avicenna, is credited with discovering the method of distillation of essential oils and contributing several authoritative texts on their properties. In the Middle Ages, European influences strengthened, with herbs and spices helping to ward off the Black Death in the fourteenth century. Further developments in phytotherapy (plant therapy) and perfumery occurred in the sixteenth century in Switzerland, France, Italy and Germany, and in the seventeenth century in Britain when Culpepper wrote his famous Herbal.

Unfortunately, several factors contributed to the decline in the use of plants in the eighteenth century. Industrialization led to greater urbanization where people had little access to land for cultivating herbs. The chemical and pharmaceutical sciences were also developing although, ironically, the very drugs which were eventually manufactured synthetically originated from plant substances—and there is a return today to searching out new drugs which can be manufactured from plants. Medicine, too, had become a male-dominated profession and, in obstetrics, the status of the midwife was at an all-time low. Plants that had previously been harvested and administered by midwives and other women who had worked as healers were now viewed with scorn and scepticism by doctors, and dismissed as witchcraft.

The decline continued in the early twentieth century; during the Second World War the acreage available for growing plants was much reduced, especially in Germany, Austria and Hungary, although, conversely, Valnet used essential oils to treat wounded soldiers in France.

The late twentieth century has seen the re-emergence of phytotherapy, both as herbal medicine and for aromatherapy. As mentioned above, Gattefosse, a chemist, is reputed to be the modern pioneer of aromatherapy for medicinal purposes; in the 1950s in England, Marguerite Maury, a biochemist, explored the external use of essential oils, particularly for massage and cosmetic purposes. Dr Jean Valnet, now in his seventies, is probably the most noted and respected contemporary authority, who has advocated widespread use of essential oils, specifically by gastrointestinal administration. Interestingly, he does not believe that aromatherapists need to be medically qualified, and he rarely uses massage as a method of administration—and then only if the therapist wears rubber gloves to avoid skin irritation (Scott, 1993).

Science and art

Aromatherapy has now developed into a profession encompassing many different specialities with a range from the totally scientific to the truly artistic. In between the two extremes is a 'grey' area of art and science combined. Tisserand (1993) classifies these as medical aromatherapy (herbal medicine and medical science); 'nursing' aromatherapy (nursing and holistic principles); aesthetic aromatherapy (bodywork, counselling and aesthetics); psychoaromatherapy (perfumery and olfaction research); and the 'essential back-up services' of chemical analysis, plant cultivation and oil extraction. While, as midwives, we are primarily concerned with medical and nursing (in its widest sense) aromatherapy, we cannot omit an investigation of the other components of aromatherapy, all of which impinge on our understanding of this increasingly highly developed science and art.

The science of aromatherapy

Science is defined as the 'coordinated knowledge of the operation of general laws especially as obtained and tested through scientific method' in *Longman's Dictionary* (1982), and aromatherapists have gradually come to recognize the need for scientific study of the subject. Penoel (1994) identifies the disciplines involved in the science of aromatherapy as physics, biophysics, chemistry, biochemistry, botany, pharmacology, toxicology, bacteriology, psychophysiology and others.

Essential oils are highly concentrated volatile substances extracted from different parts of numerous plants, and in the science of aromatherapy are perceived as 'matter'. The term aromatherapy could be considered to undermine its scientific nature, for it is the chemical constituents of the essential oils that give them their therapeutic properties. More than this, it is the interaction of the essential oils with the human body, and the way in which that interaction takes place, that enables them to be used for medicinal purposes, or renders them potentially toxic when misused or abused.

The Single European Market has posed difficulties for complementary therapists in some countries. France and Germany, for example, do not allow the practice of any 'therapy' by anyone other than a qualified medical practitioner, or under medical supervision—the word 'therapy' implying diagnosis of a condition and subsequent prescription of treatment. A meeting in 1992 of European aromatherapists and essential oil suppliers discussed at length possible new terminology to overcome this barrier to non-medical aromatherapy, and eventually decided on the term 'aromatology' (Price, 1992). It was considered that this signified the 'study of smell' which would differentiate between treatment with herbal remedies (phytotherapy) and essential oils. (There is a degree of overlap between herbal medicine and aromatherapy but different plant constituents are used in different ways.)

The term aromatology seemed to place a greater emphasis on research and scientific demonstration of the effectiveness and modes of action of essential oils. Anecdotal evidence abounds in aromatherapy, but this takes for granted the assumed efficacy of the essential oils and does not attempt to address the question of how or why they work. Balacs (1991a) emphasizes the need for extensive research into 'oil pharmacology' to avoid exposing clients to unnecessary risks, for example oils being administered in excessively high doses or the use of oils that may interact with pharmaceutical drugs being taken contemporaneously.

Claims are made for essential oils based on available knowledge about the chemical constituents, but many suggestions for possible uses of a particular essential oil are unsubstantiated. This is especially so when discussing which oils may or may not be used in pregnancy, for no authority as yet seems prepared to commit themselves to a definitive list.

The need for research   Kirk-Smith and Stretch (1994) stress the need for and the value of research in evaluating aromatherapy practice. They pose three questions that should be asked when considering research into the clinical uses of essential oils:

1   Do they work?
2   If so, how and by what mechanism?
3   How can practice be improved by this knowledge?

These authors believe that attempting to discover the answers to the second and third questions is inappropriate until there is definite evidence that essential oils do have an effect, and they liken this to investigating elements of life on another planet before it is known whether the planet actually exists.

Research in aromatherapy, as in other complementary therapies, may be in the form of comparing the treatment under investigation with another strategy—another essential oil for the same condition—or with no treatment at all. Orthodox healthcare practitioners may alternatively wish to compare the use of an essential oil with the current conventional therapy.

In midwifery there has been little research involving the administration of essential oils, and that which has been undertaken has been based on the premise that any oils used in pregnancy or labour are generally considered to be safe because there is no documented evidence to the contrary. Trials on the potential teratogenic or abortifacient effects of essential oils have been carried out only on animals, and the huge ethical problems of researching the administration of essential oils to pregnant women means that there is a dearth of knowledge on the subject.

Pharmaceutical companies spend many years and a great deal of money on researching new drugs, and must demonstrate beyond doubt that their products are safe to be given to the public. Granted, time and expense are in their financial interest if they are eventually able to market the drug, but there are occasions when unforeseen consequences occur during testing and all development has to be abandoned.

However, this is not a viable option for aromatherapy. First, the costs would be prohibitive, and, in any case, only a small proportion of essential oil production is intended for clinical aromatherapy. Second, it is not possible to patent a natural product so there is no incentive for individual companies to undertake the research with its accompanying expense. Third, researching each oil would take an inordinate amount of time, during which period it would be necessary to withdraw the oils from public use.

The status of aromatherapy

The status of aromatherapy was, in fact, a component of the debate in 1994–1995 as a result of the threat to herbal medicines from the European Community. In England and Wales, herbal medicines have been exempt from licensing, under section 12 of the Medicines Act 1968, and from the public health safeguards that pertain to drugs, under section 56. This differs from Europe, where Napoleonic law demands that any 'industrial product' that can be used for therapeutic purposes must comply with regulations in the same manner as pharmaceutical preparations.

In October 1994 complementary practitioners became aware that, in order to conform, the British government intended to amend the law without debate, and to remove the exemptions that herbal medicines had hitherto enjoyed. A massive nationwide campaign by practitioners, producers and consumers ensued, which resulted in the Department of Health announcing that the exemption from product licensing requirements of herbal medicines would remain. Although aromatherapy products had not originally been specified in the amendment to the law, the deluge of correspondence from concerned aromatherapists prompted the Medicines Control Agency to consider its position. Eventually it was confirmed that aromatherapy products retailed in Britain would continue to be exempt from regulations, as long as no claims for therapeutic effects were made; essential oils would also remain exempt from licensing, unless administered internally—new legislation came into force in January 1995. There are still, however, some concerns about the future of aromatherapy.

Unlike drugs, there has not been, until now, any mechanism for central recording of side-effects from essential oils. However, in 1994 the European Biomedical and Health Research programme awarded a grant to the European Scientific Cooperative on Phytotherapy (ESCOP), under the direction of Simon Mills from the University of Exeter's Centre for Complementary Health Studies. The purpose of the grant is to enable the group to undertake a multicentre study on European standards for the safe and effective use of phytomedicines, part of which will involve the establishment of a pharmacovigilance project (Farrell, 1994b).

Education and training

It is also vital that, to improve the credibility of a system of care that deals with people's health, appropriate educational programmes are developed. The choice of courses for anyone wishing to undertake aromatherapy training is vast, and making a decision is difficult. Attempts to regulate training standards have been made by a joining of forces of the major aromatherapy bodies into the Aromatherapy Organisations Council (AOC), which devised minimum criteria for training with effect from January 1994. It is, however, considered by some authorities that these requirements do not go far enough in ensuring high-quality educational programmes, and some internationally renowned, reputable schools of aromatherapy have developed intensive modular programmes that surpass the minimum level. National regulation of all complementary therapies is desirable and the Health Care Sector of the Care Sector Consortium is initiating work to develop standards for complementary therapy. In late 1994 a project group was established to focus initially on standards for aromatherapy, homoeopathy, reflexology and hypnotherapy. It is expected that this work will be completed by 1997–1998. Many therapies are considering standards based on National Vocational Qualifications, but it will be the responsibility of each discipline to decide whether this is the most appropriate route for working towards a common core curriculum for complementary medicine.

For professionals working in conventional health care, much of this debate could be considered irrelevant. Educational developments within aromatherapy and other complementary therapies have evolved in an attempt to improve the status of the therapy and its practitioners, and as a result of national and international politics. Standardization of training and regulation of practice have become necessary—and desirable—in order to protect the public. Ongoing periodical refreshment and updating is seen as a means of preventing complacency, and of reflecting on and learning from previous experiences.

None of this is new to midwives, nurses or health visitors, whose initial preparation for registration, subsequent clinical practice and ongoing education are nationally regulated and monitored. Unless a midwife wishes to practise aromatherapy privately, independently of midwifery duties, she does not necessarily have to be qualified as an aromatherapist. The UK Central Council's document *The Scope of Professional Practice* (1992a) facilitates, rather than restricts, the acquisition of new skills and knowledge, so long as they are in the best interests of patients and clients, in response to their needs and do not fragment or compromise existing aspects of professional care. Individuals are personally accountable for their practice and must recognize the boundaries within which they work, including their own limitations (see also section on Accountability below).

The art of aromatherapy

Art is defined as 'a skill acquired by experience, study or observation; the conscious use of skill and creative imagination especially in the production of aesthetic objects' in *Longman's Dictionary* (1982). Penoel (1994) suggests that, in the art of aromatherapy, essential oils are seen as a 'whole', a life force inside the plant which is 'capable of exerting a deep influence on the many levels of human beings'. Tisserand (1992) likens essential oils to the blood of a person, being whole organic substances within the plant. He states:

> *Like blood they will die (lose their life force) if they are not properly preserved. Like blood they incorporate the characteristics of the body (plant) from which they come. They are like the personality, or spirit, of the plant. The essence is the most ethereal and subtle part of the plant.*

Tisserand writes of the qualities or vibrations of essential oils and the need for therapists to recognize the correlation between them and other living organisms, i.e. the human body, by refining their intuitive feelings. Much of aromatherapy is about knowing what feels right, for the client and for the practitioner; it is about individualizing care, nurturing, giving and receiving. Whereas drugs may merely suppress symptoms, there is a failure, in Western orthodox medicine, to recognize that 'illness' is the way in which the human body attempts to return to a state of harmony. Page (1994) writes of the 'message' of disease, as being 'just another manifestation of life, representing a time for change and opportunities for soul growth'. Essential oils, used correctly, work in harmony with the body, balancing it and encouraging healing to take place where necessary, without the 'violent, calculated, impersonal action' of pharmaceutical drugs.

Essential oils work at more than a simple physical level. The aromas pervade our whole being and are transported via nerves to the limbic system of the brain, where they can act on our emotions and psychological state. When essential oils are administered in the form of massage, this adds to the feeling of nurturing and will also affect our sense of wellbeing. An acknowledgement that 'good health' is not only about physical health but also about emotional and spiritual health is vitally important, and is a concept that many professionals working in conventional health care are only slowly coming to accept.

The power of aromas

The sense of smell is the most powerful sense of all, with the memory of smell being lifelong, although in the Western world it is an unsophisticated and poorly developed sense in many people. John Stephen (1994), a creative perfumer, believes that

> *it is a tragedy of our educational system that we are not taught to express ourselves in olfactory terms at an early age, in the same way that we are*

taught to do so with sight, music or tastes. The result is an olfactory vocabulary which consists of little more than 'light/heavy' and 'sweet/dry'—neither of which are very useful in describing odours!

Van Toller (Harding, 1994a) states that this inability to verbalize an odour is due, physiologically, to olfaction being dealt with in the limbic system of the brain, which is external to the cortex from which speech is derived. However, there is no difficulty in responding to an aroma, whether pleasant or distasteful, as the limbic system, originally known as the 'rhinencephalon or nose brain' is the seat of emotional and motivational behaviour.

In some cultures, such as that of the Argentinian Andean people, who are descended from the Inca, the language of olfaction is far more specific, with numerous words to describe different types of odour, and distinctions are made between the verbs for inhaling and emitting odours (Classen and Howes, 1993). The South American shamans (medicine men) today still prescribe plant aromas to alter the body odour of an ill person, and thereby transform their 'aura', in the belief that a strong aura will keep away bad spirits (Lawless, 1994).

Harding (1994b) writes of the 'scent trail' which everyone of us follows every day; of how odours invade our consciousness and add colour and dimension to our interpretation of life around us. The sense of smell helps to stimulate appetite, to inform us when food is bad or when noxious substances are in the atmosphere; anosmics have been found to lose interest in food because their taste buds are not influenced by odour. Aromas from the past can be remembered, and evoke associated memories. A personal example of the author relates to severe gestational sickness exacerbated by the smell of a particular brand of washing powder, which even today, 6 years later, reproduces the same feeling of nausea.

An American survey by Hirsch (1992a) demonstrated a difference in the odours that evoke a feeling of nostalgia, depending on the age of the person. People born before 1930 were found to favour smells such as roses, lilies, violets, attics, cut grass, meadows, fresh air, burning leaves and tweed. Those born between 1930 and 1980 preferred airplane fuel, Play-Doh, suntan oil, baby aspirin, hair spray, cocoa puffs—and marijuana, amongst other things. Hirsch postulated that in 50 years' time nostalgia will be evoked by synthetic chemical odours, but asks whether this will lead to a reduced appreciation of the natural environment.

Women, apparently, have greater sensitivity to aromas than men, with the sense of smell being strongest at ovulation (Hirsch, 1992a).

Babies, too, are receptive to odours and have been shown to respond to the smell of their own mother, particularly before natural odours are washed away (Varendi *et al.*, 1994); this may be a survival factor. Investigations by Sullivan and co-workers (1991) suggest also that olfactory associations are learnt by neonates within the first 48 hours of life.

Smokers find that their olfactory sensitivity is reduced, which in turn affects their sense of taste. Hirsch (1992b) suggests that 'more than 90 per cent of what we perceive to be taste is actually smell'.

In his investigations into olfaction, Hirsch (1992b) found that loss of the sense of smell can be due to diverse aetiology, including oestrogen-dependent breast cancer, possibly as a result of hypothalamic involvement; head injury; surgical side-effects; various cerebral and endocrine conditions; vitamin A deficiency; acute viral hepatitis; and nasal obstruction. Zinc supplements are being considered as a possible treatment for some of these causes, as many anosmics are found to be zinc deficient.

The human body emits a variety of odours. Pheromones, for example, are steroidal compounds secreted via the apocrine glands, found particularly in the axillae. The concentration of pheromones increases during sexual arousal, and pheromones are thought to play a part in the attraction of one person for another. Most cultures, throughout time, have used aromatic substances either to enhance or to mask natural odours. Pomanders of oranges stuck with cloves were carried by the wealthy during the time of the Great Plague; the fresh clean smell of rose petals used for confetti at weddings symbolizes the start of a new relationship; the ancient Egyptian courtiers used aromatic head cones to perfume the hair.

The importance of smell and its effect on mood are increasingly being recognized. Children with learning difficulties can be calmed by entering a Snoezelen room in which various ways of stimulating the senses, including olfaction, are employed. A trial in Australia, in which final demand bills were impregnated with a musky odour, reminiscent of powerful assertive men, found that debtors were much more likely to pay promptly (Anonymous, 1991). In Indiana, men found guilty of drink-driving offences are sentenced to home detention and it is stipulated that they must not drink alcohol. An alcohol sensor in the mouthpiece of the telephone enables probation officers to detect whether or not the man has been drinking; three positive calls may result in a prison sentence (Anonymous, 1994a). Dispersal of a relaxing aroma in the slot machines in Las Vegas has been found to increase gamblers' spending, with an estimated increase in revenue of £750 million a year if the procedure is introduced permanently (Anonymous, 1992).

Corporate identities may, in the future, include a company aroma that can be used for stationery; supermarkets are considering the use of aromas to encourage buying; (Anonymous, 1992; Renn, 1994); environmental fragrancing of offices and factories is already in use in Japan, and has been found to reduce computer operator errors when piped into their work areas (Renn, 1994); some schools are using fragrances to help children relax yet stimulate them to learn (Anonymous, 1993a; Maclean, 1993); and perfumed petrol has been successfully piloted in France (Anonymous, 1994b).

The power of human touch

The use of essential oils with massage is the commonest and arguably the most pleasant method of administration and offers clients legitimate human touch which enables them to relax physically and emotionally. So much of our touch in midwifery is purely functional, as it is in everyday life. The British, in particular, recognize and respect personal space to the extent that touching others is restricted to shaking hands in most situations. One trial of 250 students between the ages of 18 and 22 found that the amount of non-sexual touching of others was significantly lower than that in a similar trial of American students in the 1960s (Cripps, 1994). (Interestingly, sexual touching had increased despite the original trial being conducted at a time of so-called sexual liberation, and the replication being undertaken after the advent of acquired immune deficiency syndrome.) The reduction in the amount of touch generally may be related also to the rise in crimes against the person, particularly physical and sexual abuse of women and children, which, to avoid being misconstrued, has led to a literal distancing between people. A metaphorical distancing is also perhaps present in the hectic lifestyles we lead, resulting in less communication. Unfortunately, too, massage gained the stigma of the backstreet parlour with all its sexual implications, which has taken a long time to dispel. This has meant an uphill struggle for the many reputable practitioners in private practice, although, conversely, the incorporation of these therapies into some areas of the National Health Service (NHS) may appear to offer universal credibility irrespective of qualifications, experience or motive.

There is, in all of us, a need to be touched, which often goes unfulfilled. Infants are most likely to be touched, although this has only been the case since the policy of not handling babies was changed in the 1930s. Before this, in the early twentieth and late nineteenth centuries, over 50% of infant deaths in America were due to marasmus or 'infantile atrophy'—a lack of physical contact (Montagu, 1986).

Children are far more readily touched by their parents, although the amount of contact declines from the age of about 7 years, especially in boys. Adults in many Western cultures reserve physical contact for functional activities or for intimate relationships. The elderly are least likely to receive touch, partly as they may have lost a partner, and partly due to cultural attitudes towards the geriatric population.

Denholm (1992) suggested that people are afraid to use touch. This may be due to our innate fear of rejection, or it may be related to sexuality. It is possible that the desire for physical contact may be suppressed in case it is misunderstood, or because they fear intimacy.

Many people find it difficult to differentiate between sexuality and sensuality—aromatherapy, of course, is about sensuality, an arousal of the senses, particularly of smell and touch. Touch is about communication: we use it to communicate care and concern, to relieve pain by 'rubbing it better', to relax and to reassure. Midwives are actively involved every day in touching mothers (despite a trend towards the 'hands-off' approach), but just how much of our touch is truly nurturing rather than functional? On the other hand, midwives should be especially suited to using massage and touch. They have already learnt to 'see with their fingertips' when performing examinations per abdomen and per vaginam, and should be able to develop this sense further, learning to receive and interpret tactile information obtained from a client during massage.

Consider the language of touch in use every day. We talk of 'keeping in touch', of being 'touchy' or of being 'touched' emotionally, but there is a disparity between our vocabulary and our actions. There is no doubt, however, that touch provokes a variety of emotions, and is necessary to survival.

Professional issues for midwives

Midwives are in an invaluable position to investigate the benefits and possible dangers of aromatherapy and to encourage their use for clients. This has to be balanced against other priorities of care, especially with the constraints of time and staffing levels. Some members of the maternity services who are sceptical of the values and wary of the safety of essential oils raise these issues as a means of obstructing the implementation of aromatherapy and other complementary therapies. One of their arguments commonly is that of the financial costs of implementing aromatherapy into current practice. This is not only the costs of the oils but also the major expense of training and then of the time spent in administering essential oils.

However, once the initial costs of setting up the service, with planning meetings, staff training and purchasing the oils, have been accounted for, the use of aromatherapy does not have to add to the financial burdens of today's health service. Indeed, research with elderly patients has demonstrated considerable savings in the cost of night sedation by administering essential oil of lavender via inhalation (Hardy, 1991; Henry *et al.*, 1994).

Sources of funding other than the normal departmental budget can also be found. For example, a stress–relieving massage service for staff was set up in one unit (Lewis, 1995). Midwives qualified in massage, aromatherapy and reflexology were allowed to use on–duty time to provide the service for which staff paid a nominal fee, and the profit was used to purchase essential oils for the mothers. Donations from grateful parents could be accumulated for the same purpose; in units where transcutaneous electrical nerve stimulation (TENS) machines are loaned out to mothers prior to labour, a deposit could be charged, and experience indicates that there will probably be occasions when parents do not wish their deposit to be returned. Other fundraising activities such as boot fairs may also elicit sufficient monies to establish the service. With careful planning there are ways in which essential oils could be incorporated into client care, either in the hospital or in the home, without incurring unmanageable additional costs.

Midwives are in an even more enviable situation than many nurses for they deal in the main with healthy women. This means that the mother could administer essential oils to herself or persuade other family members to do so. Time can also be saved by adding oils to the bathwater or on a tissue rather than in a massage, or encouraging the partner to rub oil into the mother, especially during labour. Herbal teas can be prepared to obtain small amounts of the therapeutic properties, especially in pregnancy when smaller doses are necessary. The relatively new phenomenon of environmental fragrancing has also been introduced into some American hospitals, using essential oils which will produce the desired effect, e.g. calming, sedating, refreshing, uplifting (Steele, 1992).

This latter method of administration does pose a dilemma for, if essential oils are used for therapeutic reasons, they should be prescribed individually. Dissemination of aromas around a communal area of a hospital without the informed consent of everyone in that area (including staff and all visitors) could lead to potential ethicolegal difficulties. An alternative would be to use a small diffuser or add the essential oils to an inhalation apparatus or simply to a tissue; baths, footbaths or bidets, compresses and herbal teas are other means of using the oils for individuals.

The midwife may be faced with other professional problems in relation to aromatherapy. For example, a mother may arrive in the delivery suite with her own box of essential oils for self-administration during labour. If the midwife becomes aware of this, the responsibility to act on that knowledge now rests with the midwife. If she has only a superficial knowledge of aromatherapy she should inform the mother that she is unable to advise her on the correct use of the oils and that the mother must take responsibility herself for whatever she chooses to use. The midwife should record this in the notes, and also attempt to seek the advice of an aromatherapy expert for further information, in accordance with the *Midwife's Code of Practice* (UK Central Council, 1994).

An additional difficulty can occur when problems arise for which the mother in labour wishes to administer essential oils. An example of this would be a sudden rise in blood pressure requiring anti-hypertensive medication, but for which the mother wanted to use an essential oil such as ylang ylang. A combination of the two substances could result in severe hypotension with its subsequent effects on the mother, fetus and progress of labour.

Within midwifery there are many conditions that can be treated with essential oils, although their potential relative toxicity to the mother, fetus or newborn must be considered. Many essential oils are contraindicated during pregnancy or breastfeeding, and indeed some authorities feel that their use at this time is so questionable that almost all essential oils should be restricted (Ryman, 1991, p. 28). One could ask whether it is ethical to administer essential oils at all if there is so much controversy amongst aromatherapy experts. Midwives need to make themselves aware of oils that are definitely contraindicated in pregnancy, those that have a limited use for identified conditions and those that can be administered safely, albeit in lower dilution than normal. To understand the reasons for these restrictions, midwives need to know how essential oils work and the possible consequences of misuse in pregnancy.

Accountability

Midwives must abide by the publications of the United Kingdom Central Council (UKCC) which relate to the use of complementary therapies and the acquisition of new skills. The *Midwife's Code of Practice* (UKCC, 1994) acknowledges that certain new skills may become integral to the roles of all midwives, whereas other aspects, including aromatherapy, may be incorporated into the roles of a few specialist midwives. Like the *Standards for the Administration of Medicines* (UKCC, 1992b), the *Midwife's Code* emphasizes the need for sound contemporary knowledge, client consent and their right to self-administer substances such as essential oils, or to refer to a complementary practitioner. Midwives who are unsure about the effects of particular essential oils or their interaction with medication should contact the relevant expert practitioner. All midwives must ensure that they have received adequate and appropriate training to justify their actions, and need to be mindful of their own Code of Practice (UKCC, 1994) and the general *Code of Conduct for Nurses, Midwives and Health Visitors* (UKCC, 1992c). The midwife who wishes to utilize aromatherapy in her practice must be able to demonstrate that her knowledge and skills are as good as the scientific evidence available. Essential oils should be treated with the same respect accorded to drugs, and midwives must abide by the standards laid down for the administration of medicines (UKCC, 1992b).

Midwives and doctors cannot, in the best interests of their clients, afford to be complacent, antagonistic or confrontational about complementary therapies. It is far preferable that the professions accept, at the very least, that clients wish to use 'alternatives' and that we have much to learn from both complementary practitioners and consumers. Anticipation of demand from mothers, even in areas where there has hitherto been none, should prompt active, constructive, multidisciplinary discussion about the issues of concern to the maternity care team. These can then be resolved or a compromise reached in advance of parents' demands. As more women become interested and involved in aromatherapy, it may become necessary to ask routine questions at booking and at the onset of labour about whether a mother is using any essential oils. This could easily be included in the questions on medication. A policy of openness about clients' uses of all complementary therapies will facilitate communication between mothers and their carers before a potentially dangerous situation develops.

Religious conflicts   Some women may reject aromatherapy or other complementary therapies because of their religious beliefs, and these should, of course, be respected. However, their arguments are often founded on lack of knowledge and it may be useful here to consider the issue.

Linda North (1994) wrote in distress about the reaction of her local clergyman to an advertisement for aromatherapy in the Parish magazine. Apparently he was so incensed that he instigated amongst the parishioners a campaign against aromatherapy in general and against the therapist in particular. Sadly this is not an isolated case, and many Christians are concerned about what they see as 'New Age' therapies which incorporate many eastern concepts such as Yin and Yang, aura detection and magic.

In response, it may be appropriate to focus on the scientific element of aromatherapy, highlighting the similarities with modern pharmaceuticals. Many of the chemical constituents of essential oils are used for proven therapeutic purposes—and plant medicines were the precursors of modern-day drugs. Midwives will be aware that ergometrine was developed from the ergot fungus which was found to grow on rye, and that the contraceptive pill originated from the yam.

The essential oils are extracted from the plants and are not manipulated in any way, unlike homoeopathic remedies which require diluting and succussing (shaking) to activate the therapeutic energy, which is, as yet, not fully proven.

The use of plants as medicines stretches back to biblical times, and essential oils were used for healing, cleansing and anointing; indeed, the practice of some Christian religions still involves the burning of incense during periods of worship. Page (1994) stressed the need to 'break down the barriers which exist between religion, philosophy, psychology and medicine and (to) realise that they each represent only part of the whole picture' (pp. 19–21).

The administration of essential oils should be viewed as another means of assisting people to 'feel good' about themselves, but should not be forced on to them if they have reservations. Until more research is undertaken and there is an increase in understanding and acceptance of aromatherapy amongst conventional health profesionals (especially doctors) sceptics and those who see aromatherapy as 'New Age' will not be convinced.

Protocols   All maternity service areas should consider the need to develop protocols regarding complementary therapies and/or aromatherapy in particular. The generally fit healthy young women who are our customers are possibly among the most likely NHS users to be interested in essential oils. Unit or district policies or protocols will serve to safeguard both the health of the women and the professional integrity of the midwifery staff.

It may be feasible to gather together a small group of interested staff to explore the issues and produce a draft policy which could then be presented for discussion at one of the unit liaison meetings.

Aspects for consideration by the group might be:

1   A policy for staff to deal with visiting complementary practitioners.
2   An action plan for women who wish to self-administer remedies.
3   A protocol for staff using aromatherapy or any other complementary therapy within their practice.

Visiting therapists   An aromatherapist who is not a member of the maternity staff should be made aware from the outset that the midwife and/or consultant obstetrician maintains overall responsibility for the mother's care during this period, so that an atmosphere of mutual cooperation and teamwork can be engendered wherever possible. Any essential oils adminstered to the mother, especially during the acute period of labour and delivery, should be with the knowledge and consent of the midwife; this particularly applies to emergency situations or at any time when medications are being given. For example, if a woman has a long difficult labour because of a posterior position of the fetal occiput, there may come a time when she requests additional analgesia in the form of epidural anaesthesia. The attending aromatherapist may have been using a blend of oils for pain relief which includes lavender, but this should be eliminated once the epidural is *in situ*, for the combined hypotensive effects of the bupivacaine and the lavender could adversely influence the mother's blood pressure to such an extent that fetal oxygenation is compromised.

The midwife or unit manager should ensure that the visiting therapist has adequate and up-to-date insurance to practise, to avoid the possibility of claims for negligence later being made against the health authority. The mother should be advised to check that the therapist has adequate experience of caring for childbearing women.

In units where complementary therapists are welcomed, some practitioners may become regular visitors and can be consulted as a resource. If mothers request advice about or referral to an aromatherapist, it may be appropriate to recommend one of these 'regulars' rather than leave to chance the selection of an aromatherapist without adequate experience by mothers perusing the 'Yellow Pages'. However, midwives should be cautious about referring women to specific practitioners unless they are certain that they are experts in the field.

Women self-administering essential oils

Women have a right to administer substances such as essential oils to themselves, and the views of midwives should not prove an obstacle to them doing so. However, it is important that the attending midwife is aware of what is being used, so, to avoid the mother feeling she must use them clandestinely, she should be asked on admission whether or not she wishes to administer them.

Midwives should advise women of the need to consider carefully what they use and how much; even those staff who know none of the details of individual essential oils should be aware that they are contraindicated in the first trimester and that there are many oils that should not be administered at all during pregnancy. The production of a leaflet could be considered, which warns mothers of some of the potential dangers, without worrying those who may already have used oils in pregnancy.

Midwives using essential oils within their own practice

Midwives who have received training and education in the use of aromatherapy for childbearing women may be able to administer oils to their clients. It must be stressed, however, that it is not professionally acceptable merely to commence using the oils during their midwifery duties, if managers and supervisors have not agreed. This author has been concerned while lecturing around the country that some midwives seem not to understand issues of professional accountability and fail to recognize that they are intended not only as a protection for the public, but also for the practitioner.

Midwives who are qualified aromatherapists must learn to differentiate between the two roles. The midwife who has a private aromatherapy practice is working as a member of the complementary therapy professions and should not undertake midwifery responsibilities, e.g. abdominal examination, when seeing clients who happen to be pregnant. Independent midwives may use aromatherapy or any other complementary therapy within their practice so long as they comply with the requirements of the UK Central Council: the *Midwives' Code of Practice* (UKCC, 1994), *The*

Scope of Professional Practice (UKCC, 1992a) and the *Standards for the Administration of Medicines* (UKCC, 1992b). The midwife carrying out normal antenatal, intrapartum and puerperal care who is employed in a NHS or private maternity unit may use aromatherapy only with the knowledge and approval of managers and supervisors.

Managers are advised to facilitate the development of policies and protocols which record in detail the factors which they consider important. The following may be considered as necessary inclusions.

Training   The type of aromatherapy training accepted may be any course approved by one of the aromatherapy organizations, although individual courses may vary and may not focus specifically on pregnancy-related issues. Alternatively, in-house training in a limited number of essential oils directly relevant to the client group may be favoured.

Approved staff   Staff approved to use aromatherapy in their practice should be named; it may be necessary to identify those who are fully qualified aromatherapists and those who have undertaken a short course as suggested above. Some units may wish to develop the skills of a few of the healthcare assistants, who could undertake a short National Vocational Qualification style of training in the administration of massage. A qualified midwife-aromatherapist would need to oversee their work, prescribe treatments and dispense the oils, but the actual administration, especially where this is via massage, could quite feasibly be carried out by the healthcare assistants. This would have the benefit of enabling an aromatherapy service to be established whilst conserving midwifery time, thus making cost-effective use of the staff available.

Selection of essential oils   Although midwife-aromatherapists will technically be able to use any essential oil considered safe for the client group, managers may want to specify a limited selection for use within the unit, in an attempt to monitor the effects and retain control of the situation. It may also be necessary to consider whether to restrict the number of essential oils in a blend. Using them singly will enable identification of the causes of side-effects, whereas a blend of more than one essential oil will act synergistically (see Chapter 6). Decisions may be made also about which base oil is to be used; this may be influenced by cost, if nothing else.

Dosage   This would include the permitted doses of blends and the amount any one mother may receive each day. For instance, where lavender oil is used for perineal care, two 5-ml doses of 2 per cent lavender in base oil, added to the bath water, may be approved as the total daily dose. The doses should be written on the label of the bottle.

Route of administration   This may alter according to the symptom being treated. For instance, constipation may be resolved by abdominal massage, whereas perineal trauma may be eased by putting essential oils into the bath or bidet, or chest infections may require inhalations. Health and safety regulations may preclude certain methods of administration such as vaporization using a candle, although this author has been horrified to learn that this is not uncommon practice in some general wards.

Client selection   This would include categories of women who may or may not be treated with essential oils by midwives; for example, it may be considered best only to treat women less than gravida four, who have a singleton pregnancy, with a cephalic presentation in the last trimester, and who are normotensive (although this latter factor is debatable as essential oils can be beneficial in lowering or raising blood pressure).

Conditions   Conditions that may be treated include constipation, insomnia, stress, pain relief in labour, perineal care, oedema: it is preferable to specify certain conditions, especially when the service is being developed, rather than encourage midwives to treat any condition that may respond to aromatherapy. Dealing with the physiological symptoms of pregnancy, labour and the puerperium is a normal part of the midwife's role and would be the most appropriate starting point.

Restrictions   This would outline conditions in which aromatherapy is contraindicated locally: for example, some units may not allow women to be treated at all antenatally in the light of the controversy surrounding safe use of essential oils at this time, preferring to restrict use to labour and the puerperium. Women with major medical or obstetric problems may be included on this list, or may receive aromatherapy only after medical consultation. Paediatric medical staff may wish to confine the use of massage to healthy neonates and to specify that only base oils are used, rather than essential oils.

Blending This would name the staff responsible for blending essential and base oils. This may be one or two named midwives, preferably who are qualified aromatherapists, rather than permitting each member of staff to blend their own oils before administration. A stock can be made available from which all other staff on the 'approved list' dispense the ready-blended oil as required.

Approved documentation It will need to be decided whether the consent obtained from the client is to be recorded in writing or can be accepted verbally. Records of the essential oils administered must be maintained either in the normal midwifery records or the main notes, if these are different, or on a separate form. Although it is unlikely that obstetricians will wish to sign 'standing orders' for the actual oils, as they are not appropriately qualified to do so, it may be pertinent to obtain 'blanket' approval for the use of aromatherapy within the unit, in accordance with locally defined policies.

PART 1

The Science of Aromatherapy

in Midwifery Practice

Chapter 2

Extraction, Quality and Storage of Essential Oils

Extraction of essential oils from plants

Essential oils are the highly volatile fluid constituents in plants, usually found in tiny droplets in the veins, glands, glandular hairs and sacs. Their function in the plant is to act as regulators, hormones and catalysts, and to assist the plant in adapting to environments that would normally be stressful, with a consequent increase in growth. Essential oils also act as a protection for the plant against diseases, parasites and, in very hot areas, the sun. Some essential oils help to attract insects for pollination and may work as natural weedkillers on the surrounding soil. They are often coloured, do not dissolve in water but mix well in vegetable oils, fats and waxes, and fairly well in alcohol.

Some plants yield a minute amount of essential oil compared with others; for example, over 100 kg of rose petals are required to produce just 50–80 g of the essential oil, which makes true rose oil extremely expensive (Arcier, 1992, p. 20). The chemical constituents of an individual type of essential oil can vary according to the geographical terrain and climate, the time of day and the season. An investigation into *Rosmarinus officinalis* (rosemary) demonstrated similarity of chemical components in oils obtained from Hungary and Germany, but there was an absence of camphor and borneol in the sample from England (Hethelyi *et al.*, 1987). An exploration of ten samples of rosemary from British oil producers also demonstrated considerable differences in chemical constituents and showed that rosemary was often adulterated by the addition of eucalyptus and camphor oils (Svoboda and Deans, 1990) in an attempt to replace the constituents that were missing.

Different parts of plants will produce different essential oils; for instance, from the orange tree can be extracted essential oils of orange (from the rind), neroli (from the orange blossom) and petitgrain (from the twigs). Many of the essential oils derived from culinary herbs, such as sage, rosemary and marjoram, have been extracted from the leaves. Others are extracted from the fruit, especially the citrus oils, from the flowers (neroli, camomile), seeds (carrot seed, black pepper) or the bark or inner part of a tree (sandalwood, rosewood).

The method of extraction will depend on the part of the plant from which the essential oil is derived and the difficulty in so doing. Extraction of citrus essences is a relatively simple process of expression and many readers will themselves have been able to extract the essence from an orange, merely in the act of peeling the fruit: the spurt of liquid is essence from the peel, not juice from the flesh of the orange. Most essential oils are extracted through a process of steam distillation but the opposite extreme is the complicated solvent extraction process for oils from delicate petals such as jasmine, neroli or rose, for they would be damaged both by expression or steam distillation.

Steam distillation The original process of distillation is attributed to the Arab physician Avicenna, although it is possible that the ancient Egyptians used a similar process. In principle, the procedure has changed little since its origins.

Using a specially constructed still, boiled water is turned to steam which then softens the plant tissues allowing the essential oils to escape. The essential oil vaporizes and rises to pass into the vapour pipe, where it is cooled and a mixture of oil and water is collected. This can be separated fairly easily by means of a filter system or centrifugal separator (Fig. 2.1).

The actual process of distillation is simple, although some plants have to undergo the process several times in order to obtain the full yield of essential oil. The oil producer needs skill and experience to ensure that the plants are prepared appropriately to obtain optimum yields. In some plants, such as sandalwood and cedarwood, the essential oil-containing cells are situated deep within hard tissue so that the chips of wood have to be almost powdered down to rupture

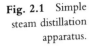

Fig. 2.1 Simple steam distillation apparatus.

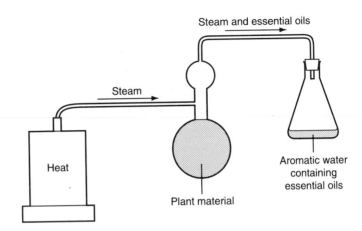

the cell walls for the essential oil to be accessed. This is known as comminution.

Timing of the extraction process is important too, as some plants need immediate distillation to avoid the essential oil being lost or destroyed, e.g. melissa. Some plants may be left to remove excess water before distillation, e.g., lavender, and others may be completely dried out, e.g. black pepper seeds.

A new method of extraction which works on a principle similar to that of a coffee percolator, called hydrodiffusion, is now being used in France and appears to produce more aromatic and highly coloured essential oils than those produced by steam distillation (Price, 1993, p. 18).

Carbon dioxide extraction An extremely expensive method of using compressed carbon dioxide as a solvent to extract the essential oils has also been available since the early 1980s, producing oils closer to those in the actual plant. Although the equipment costs several million pounds it has been used in a few units in France, Japan, Germany and America, and could be used commercially in the near future (Lavabre, 1990, p. 21) This method has the advantage of using a lower temperature so that the essential oils are not damaged by heat, and it is much quicker than steam distillation, which can take up to 48 hours to complete, with the risk of some oxidation of the essential oils.

Cold expression This process is used to extract oils from citrus fruits, although lime oil is more often distilled than expressed.

Crushing of the whole fruit followed by separation of the essential oil from the juice and peel is one method of expression. Alternatively the outer rind of the fruit may be abraded and the essence collected after centrifugal separation from the debris, a method used to obtain bergamot oil.

Expressed oils usually have a small amount of antioxidant added to them to prevent rapid deterioration, but the storage life of these oils is still fairly short, about 3 months. The essences should be stored in a cool dark place, preferably in the refrigerator as light and heat will initiate the degeneration process.

Solvent extraction The original method of extraction used for delicate flowers such as roses, jasmine or orange blossom is called enfleurage. It involved pressing the petals between layers of fat until the fat was saturated with essential oils which were then removed by distillation.

In plants where heat or water may cause damage to the essential oils, solvent extraction is now used to produce essential oils classed as absolutes or resinoids, which are highly concentrated aromatic materials. Resins are the exudates from trees which partially or totally solidify on mixing with air. Solvents such as hydrocarbons are used to extract the aromatic material from the resin; these are later filtered off and removed by distillation.

Some authorities believe that absolutes are not suitable for use in aromatherapy and should be used only in perfumery as they almost always retain some of the solvent (Lavabre, 1990, p. 19), although this should be under ten parts per thousand (Ryman, 1991, p. 10). Others suggest that they may be used for therapeutic work but that practitioners should be aware of the possible sensitivity caused by the solvent residue which may occur in some people (Price, 1993, p. 21).

Occasionally solvent extraction is preferred over steam distillation in order to produce an absolute with a different type of aroma from the essential oil. For example, the perfumery industry may use an absolute of lavender for a variety of purposes, rather than the essential oil. When an absolute is used in aromatherapy it is vital to purchase from a reputable supplier who can account for its origins, for the extra cost involved in production can lead some producers to adulterate the absolute with a cheaper essential oil or a synthetic substitute.

**Quality of
essential oils**

It is imperative when using essential oils therapeutically that they are of the highest possible quality. This is a problem, however, as the essential oil producers supply the vast majority of their oils to the perfumery and food industries with only a small proportion of business going to the aromatherapy market. Although there are obviously stringent quality controls for these other industries, they do not have the same priorities and it would be an extremely costly exercise for producers to adapt equipment and procedures for such analyses as are required by aromatherapists.

It has already been mentioned that the chemical profile of an essential oil can be affected by a variety of factors such as climate. The addition of chemical fertilizers and weedkillers can also, of course, adversely affect the plant and thus the essential oil. The only sure way to obtain the best quality oil is to find a supplier of organic essential oils, but these will be more expensive. It is true that 'you get what you pay for' in aromatherapy, but this is surely in the interests of clients receiving the oils.

It is useful here to compare essential oils to pharmacological drugs. Pharmaceutical companies apply for patents for drugs in which the active ingredients are blended to a specific 'secret'—and later, patented—recipe. Similar drugs are available in a generic form but the exact combination of chemical ingredients will differ slightly and may affect an individual differently. An example of this can be seen in the varying responses one person may have to two different brands of iron tablet.

In aromatherapy an individual essential oil is selected for its known therapeutic properties, due to the balance of chemical components. If a particular batch of essential oil lacks some of those chemicals, perhaps due to climatic conditions (essential oils are like wine, there are good years and bad years), some producers may attempt to add the missing ingredient, either from another essential oil or with a synthetic substance. It is also known that certain of the more expensive oils or absolutes are adulterated with cheaper oils which have a similar odour. For instance, rose may have rose geranium, palmarosa, lemongrass or even synthetic chemicals such as stearine or a terpenic alcohol added in an attempt to raise profits (Lavabre, 1990, p. 20).

An increasing number of essential oil suppliers now provide a written analysis of the actual oil being sold with a guarantee of quality control mechanisms. When essential oils are as pure as can be found, the therapist will in fact need to use less to achieve the same results—a little like some of the advertisements for washing-up liquid seen on television. Organic or biological essential oils are issued with a certificate of proof, although it must be recognized that, despite organic growing methods without the use of pesticides, it is still possible for the plants to have been exposed to environmental contamination outside the control of the grower, such as the Chernobyl disaster.

Analysis of essential oils

Essential oils can be analysed using a system called gas chromatography. The original process was invented in the 1920s to separate chlorophylls from plants but was not really developed further until the 1960s; by the 1980s the process had become much more sophisticated.

Chromatography in its simplest form involves the application of a thin layer of silica gel to a glass plate, to which is added, near one end of the plate, a minute amount of the substance to be analysed. The glass plate is inserted into a lidded receptacle containing a solvent which rises by capillary action up the plate. As the solvent moves up the plate, the solute (in this case, essential oils) is washed up the plate with it. The analysis depends on the fact that different solutes move upwards at different rates, thus a 'fingerprint' of an essential oil can be made. Technological advances now mean that chromatography can be performed using computerized machinery (Fig. 2.2).

Gas chromatography is similar in principle to the simple chromatography described above but uses gases instead of silica–coated plates. A modern development is the use of high-performance liquid chromatography, which may replace gas chromatography within the next 10 years.

Chromatographic analysis is undertaken when the purity of an essential oil is in question. The analysis of the oil is matched against the known profile of the named oil, and may show the presence of undesirable constituents.

A case is known to this author of a nurse who bought some 'neroli oil' from a popular high street retailer of beauty products. After advice from a friend she added a mere three drops of the oil to her bath water one evening. She sat in the bath for several minutes and then apparently 'blacked out' for a few seconds. She was eventually able to get out of the bath, and put her experience down to the bath water being too hot, although she was accustomed to having a hot bath. A few days later she tried the oil again, using only three drops in the water as before. This time she felt herself becoming lightheaded and faint, and quickly got out of the bath.

Fig 2.2 (a) Modern
chromatography
equipment.

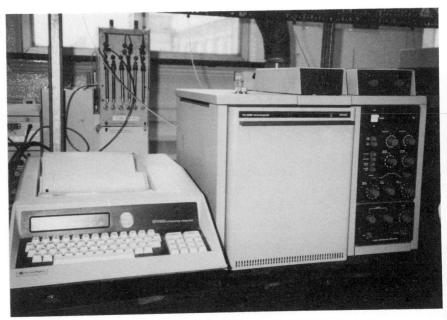

Fig 2.2 (b) High-
performance liquid
chromatography.

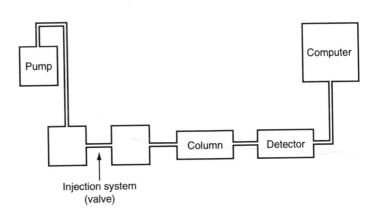

The nurse returned the oil to the shop where she had bought it and was initially met with derision until she insisted on having the oil analysed. It was only after she left the shop that it occurred to her that she should have kept some of the oil to obtain an independent analysis. Unfortunately the report returned from the supplier did not elicit any contamination of the oil. However, the important fact here is that the shop does not sell essential oils; they offer a selection of aromatic oils which smell good but are not intended for therapeutic use. Although the shop makes no claims for the oils, it is the lack of knowledge on the part of the public which leads them to believe that aromatic oils are the same as essential oils. Furthermore, this misconception is not repudiated by the retailer and adds to the lack of credibility of aromatherapy.

Storage of essential oils

Essential oils are expensive and deserve to be kept in a way that will retain their properties for as long as possible. They are also toxic when misused (i.e. overdosed), and from an accountability point of view should therefore be stored with the same regard to safety as drugs.

Physically, essential oils will deteriorate, or oxidize, when they are exposed to oxygen, light or changing temperatures. Essential oils are supplied in dark brown or blue bottles which should be stored in a cool dark place to avoid oxidation which can be caused by the ozone present in bright sunlight. The bottles should always be made of glass as plastic may act as a chemical catalyst and initiate degenerative changes; in addition, ultraviolet light from the sun, which could adversely affect the oils, will not penetrate through glass. Where bottles are supplied with a dropper, these should also be of glass. However, droppers with rubber tops should, for similar reasons, be stored separately from the essential oils.

It is better to purchase quantities that will be used up fairly quickly, rather than buying in bulk, which would be uneconomic if the oils are unused within their estimated therapeutic shelf-life. Most essential oils retain their properties for up to a year; after this time polymerization, the breaking up of double bonds in the compounds, may cause changes to occur, leaving a sediment (which will be a contaminant) in the base of the bottle. Some authorities consider that certain essential oils may keep for up to 2 or even 3 years if they are well stored (Lavabre, 1990, p. 22), but some oils such as the citrus essences are known to have a shelf-life of only 3–6 months.

Essential oils should also be kept unblended for as long as possible because once they are mixed with a carrier oil the process of oxidation will begin. This may mean that certain of the chemicals break down to form different products, thus altering the profile of the oil and its therapeutic value. Concentrated essential oils should have the lid of the bottle firmly closed and, indeed, it is good practice, especially when carrying out a full body massage, which can take over an hour, for the blended oil to be kept covered or in a container with a lid. Water will also cause oxidation, so sprays containing essential oils should be used up within a day of mixing.

To store essential oils *safely* they should be kept away from children and, in a maternity unit, in a locked cupboard or refrigerator, clearly identified. Individual bottles should be labelled with the name of the oil, and for blended oils the concentration, name of the carrier oil, date of blending and expiry, and the name of the person responsible. Ideally essential oil bottles should have an integral dropper in the neck to avoid inadvertent overdosing; recommendations on this issue are made by the Aromatherapy Organizations Council to members of the oil-producing trade. Further work does need to be done, however, on regulating the labelling of bottles of essential oils. Sadly, rare cases of near-fatal poisoning with essential oils do reach the professional press, as in the report of a child who ingested clove oil which resulted in coma, acidosis, severe hypoglycaemia, disseminated intravascular coagulation and hepatic failure. Fortunately, after intensive treatment, the child made a full recovery but the authors of the report made several recommendations about the labelling of essential oil containers (Hartnoll *et al.*, 1993). The dearth, or inaccuracy, of information given to the lay public when they purchase essential oils is deplorable, and it is not surprising that occasional reports of misuse reach the medical press, a fact that does nothing to enhance the credibility of aromatherapy as a reputable form of health care.

Chapter 3

Properties and Constituents of Essential Oils

To appreciate the scientific nature of aromatherapy it is necessary to understand some basic chemical concepts. Chemistry is the study of matter and its properties; matter is everything that has mass and occupies space. Organic chemistry is the study of chemistry in living things, i.e. plants and animals, or perhaps it could be referred to as the study of the carbon compound, for all living things contain carbon. Inorganic chemistry refers to non-living matter and is not relevant to aromatherapy.

An *element* is a chemical substance that cannot be split into simpler substances, with all the atoms in it having the same number of protons. There are 92 natural elements, including hydrogen, carbon, nitrogen and oxygen, plus some formed by nuclear reactions. Some of these elements are gases and therefore the lightest, others are solids and two are liquids; some elements are reactive, others are not.

An *atom* is the smallest particle of an element which cannot be subdivided further. An atom has a nucleus containing one or more electrically positive protons and one or more neutral neutrons. Negative electrical charges (electrons) orbit the perimeter of the atom, with usually two on the inner shell and up to eight on the outer shell of the atom. The atoms of particular elements are all identical, but those of another element are different from the first (Fig. 3.1).

Fig 3.1(a) Atoms and
elements.
(b) The water
compound.
(c) Valency of water.

(a)

Electrons
(–ve charge)

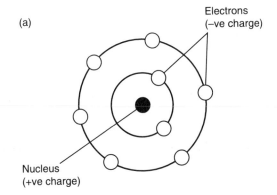

Nucleus
(+ve charge)

(b)

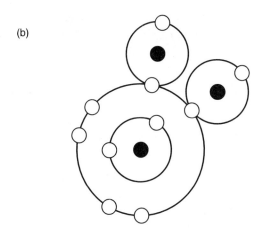

(c)

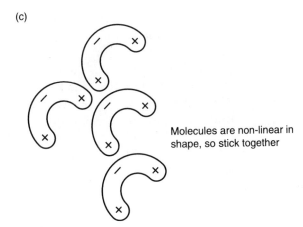

Molecules are non-linear in
shape, so stick together

Valency refers to the combining power of different elements as a result of the number of 'hooks' or 'arms' each has. Hydrogen has only one 'hook' so will bond with only one other element; therefore it is said to have a valency of 1. Oxygen has a valency of 2, so that when it combines with hydrogen both 'hooks' bond with a hydrogen element; thus $H=O=H$ or H_2O is formed, i.e. water (Fig. 3.1).

A *compound* is formed when two or more elements are attached to each other, for example the compound carbon dioxide consists of one carbon element and two oxygen elements joined together. The shape of the compound affects what that compound is able to do: one oxygen element with two hydrogen elements attached is bent, so several compounds 'stick' together as water.

A *molecule* is the smallest particle of a compound, when atoms are bonded together. Within one compound all the molecules have the same number of atoms.

When compounds are formed, all the 'hooks' of each element must be bonded to one another for the compound to be complete. Those molecules which are the most difficult to separate are the most stable, such as nitrogen in which the three 'hooks' of one molecule are securely attached to the three 'hooks' of another. This differs from hydrogen molecules with only one 'hook' each, which are easily separated and therefore unstable (Fig. 3.1).

In some compounds double bonds are formed, but these are more easily broken down by chemical processes. Many of the constituents of essential oils contain double bonds, which is why factors such as light and heat cause the oils to deteriorate. Another example is the addition of essential oils to water for sprays: it is necessary to use distilled water as the presence of chlorine in tap water adversely affects the essential oils and begins the process of oxidation. Incidentally, double bonds are partly responsible for the colours of essential oils; the colour increases as the number of double bonds increases.

A *mixture* has more than one kind of molecule within it, unlike a compound which has only one type. A mixture may be separated by various processes into its individual molecules. When compounds are submitted to physical changes, such as melting, boiling or condensing, the molecules remain unchanged, but with chemical changes, for example combustion, there are large energy changes involving heat and light which result in the molecules being changed and atoms rearranged. This can be demonstrated when 1 g of magnesium is burned: due to the addition of oxygen during burning, almost 2 g of white powder are the end-product.

Volatility refers to the fact that essential oils evaporate easily and are also flammable when they come in contact with extremes of heat; this is important when considering where to store the oils. Care must also be taken when using candle burners that the essential oils do not come into direct contact with the flame.

To smell the aroma of an essential oil, at least one molecule has to evaporate and enter the nostril. Imagine, then, the number of molecules that must be present in a few drops of essential oil which evaporate in a large room, yet can be smelt by everyone present in that room. In fact 1 ml (1 cc) of essential oil actually contains 1×10^{22} molecules, i.e. 10,000,000,000,000,000,000,000 molecules.

Constituents of essential oils

It is the chemical constituents of essential oils that give them their therapeutic properties (Table 3.1). When analysis of an essential oil is carried out a list of the main 'ingredients' is made; those in the largest proportions are usually placed at the beginning of the list, in the same way that lists of ingredients in food products are in priority order.

All essential oils are formed as the result of combinations of carbon, hydrogen and oxygen. These are the foundations of all other constituents within the oils: mono-, sesqui- and di-terpenes, alcohols, aldehydes, ketones, acids, esters, ethers, coumarins, oxides and lactones. Substances such as tannins, mucilages and flavonoids are plant constituents used therapeutically by medical herbalists but are not found in essential oils. This is partly because the extraction process usually involves the use of water, so that only small, volatile, water-insoluble substances can be isolated from the plant.

Monoterpenes Monoterpenes are made up of two chains of five carbon atoms known as isoprenes, i.e. they contain ten atoms of carbon, together with hydrogen atoms attached to the 'arms' of the atoms; they are the smallest of the terpenoid molecules. Monoterpenes occur in almost all essential oils in varying proportions, and include camphene, limonene (Fig. 3.2), myrcene, phellandrene and pinene. As can be seen, the names all end in 'ene', making them easy to identify. They are antibacterial, especially in air, and occasionally antiviral. They are stimulating and act as a mild analgesic; research by Lorenzetti et al. (1991) found that myrcene, a constituent of lemongrass oil, appears to act as a peripheral analgesic without tolerance developing after repeated administration. Monoterpenes also have expectorant properties, as has been demonstrated by Boyd and Sheppard's (1970) investigations into camphene, a major constituent of nutmeg oil. Schafer and Schafer (1981) elicited broncholytic

Table 3.1
Therapeutic properties of some phytochemicals

Chemical constituent	Functional group	Therapeutic property	Example of essential oil
Arbutin	Phenol	Diuretic Urinary antiseptic Antitussive	Marjoram
Benzoic acid	Phenol	Antifungal Choleretic	Benzoin
Bergapten	Coumarin	Photoxic	Bergamot
Bornyl acetate	Ester	Expectorant	Rosemary
Camphene	Monoterpene	Cholesterol-reducing	Nutmeg Cypress
Camphor	Ketone	Rubefacient Irritant Mild analgesic	Lavender Cinnamon
Carvacrol	Phenol	Antiseptic Antifungal Antihelmintic	Thyme Marjoram
Chamazulene	Sesquiterpene	Anti-inflammatory Antipyretic Antiphlogistic	Camomile
Cinnamic aldehyde	Aldehyde	Lacrimatory Skin irritant	Cinnamon
1.8 Cineole	Oxide	Expectorant Antihelmintic	Eucalyptus
Citral	Aldehyde	Antiseptic (5 × phenol)	Lemongrass
Farnesol	Alcohol	Antibacterial	Rose Camomile
Fenchone	Ketone	Counter-irritant	Fennel
Geraniol	Alcohol	Antiseptic (7 × phenol)	Geranium Rose
Limonene	Monoterpene	Sedative Expectorant Skin irritant	Lemon Orange Mandarin

Table 3.1 continued	Linalol	Alcohol	Antiseptic (5 × phenol)	Lavender Bergamot
	Menthol	Alcohol	Mucolytic Antipruritic Carminative Analgesic	Mint oils
	Zingiberene	Monoterpene	Carminative	Ginger

Fig 3.2 Structure of (a) limonene and (b) zingiberene.

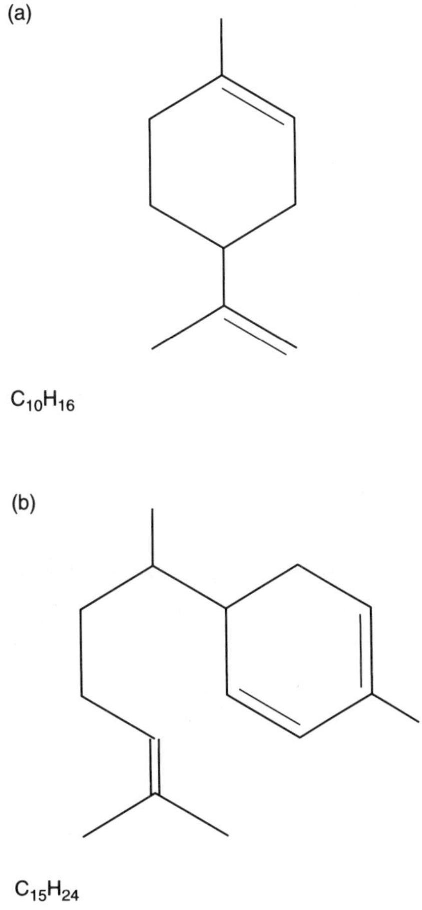

(a)

$C_{10}H_{16}$

(b)

$C_{15}H_{24}$

and secretolytic effects from an ointment containing camphene (and menthol). Monoterpenes are thought to irritate the skin in susceptible people, so should always be administered in a base oil if they are to come in contact with the skin, although Price (1993, p. 36) suggests that dextro-limonene may 'quench' the irritating effects of other constituents such as aldehyde in lemongrass oil. Monoterpenes have been found to be soluble in blood and in oil, which suggests that they will accumulate in the adipose tissues of the body. This occurs particularly when administered via the respiratory tract, as shown by Falk-Filipsson's work (1993) in which healthy men inhaled *d*-limonene in varying concentrations with a 70 per cent respiratory uptake and a long half-life. *d*-Limonene is also thought to have potential value in detoxifying chemical carcinogens as it has been found (with geraniol, in lemongrass oil) to increase the activity of glutathione *S*-transferase (a detoxifying liver enzyme) in mice (Zheng *et al.*, 1993).

Sesquiterpenes   The term sesqui means 'one and a half', and sesquiterpenes contain one and a half monoterpenes, or three isoprene units of five carbon atoms. The isoprene units may be in a long chain or in a cyclical formation, such as α-farnesene found in citronella and zingiberene in ginger oil (Fig. 3.2).

Sesquiterpenes share some similarities of action with monoterpenes, being antiseptic, antibacterial and analgesic, but they are also anti-inflammatory, antispasmodic and hypotensive, and, unlike the stimulating effects of monoterpenes, sesquiterpenes are relaxing; in addition they do not seem to be skin irritants.

Examples of sesquiterpenes include α-terpinene, β-bisabolene, farnesene and sabinene (again the names end in 'ene').

These molecules are bigger and heavier than monoterpenes and have decreased volatility; they are therefore more susceptible to oxidation by light, especially as many of them are more deeply coloured than monoterpenes. Conversely, monoterpenes are more likely to oxidize in the presence of oxygen in air, although oxygen does play a part in producing other functional groups (see below).

Diterpenes   Diterpenes consist of two monoterpenes, i.e. four isoprene units, and are found to a much lesser extent in essential oils as they are bigger, heavier, less volatile molecules. Therapeutically, diterpenes have a weak anti-infective action, being antibacterial, antiviral and antifungal in some cases; they are also slightly expectorant and are thought to balance the endocrine system.

There are also terpenoid molecules that consist of six or even eight isoprene units, but these are much too heavy to evaporate during the extraction process, and so they are not found in essential oils. This group includes steroids and some hormones.

Other constituents As discussed above, terpenes are all made up of a number of isoprene units, or multiples of *five* carbon atoms (with a minimum of two), in a *chain* (called aliphatic molecules). When *six* carbon atoms combine in a *ring* this is known as a benzene or aromatic ring, or, more commonly now, as a hydrocarbon phenyl ring. With either a chain or a ring formation, other functional groups of atoms may attach themselves to form molecules with a variety of shapes, and therefore with different therapeutic properties. Where molecules consist of only hydrogen and carbon they are called unsubstituted hydrocarbons (i.e. monoterpenes, sesquiterpenes and diterpenes), but when other functional groups attach themselves, some of the hydrogen atoms are replaced with oxygen and these are termed substituted compounds. Terpenoid alcohols, aldehydes, ketones and acids are formed when groups of atoms attach to chain molecules. Phenolic compounds are formed when these same functional groups attach to a phenyl ring, with the addition of another group of molecules called phenols.

Terpenic alcohols Terpenic alcohols are formed when an aliphatic terpene chain is joined by an unstable hydroxyl group (water molecules that have lost one of the hydrogen atoms), and may be monoterpenols, sesquiterpenols or diterpenols according to the size of the aliphatic chain to which they become attached. The suffix '-ol' is helpful in identifying the alcohols, although confusion may arise as many phenols also end in 'ol'. The change in shape that occurs as a result of the addition of the hydroxyl group will denote the characteristics, both chemical and therapeutic, of the individual compound, with some remaining in a linear chain and others becoming cyclic. The aroma of essential oils with a high proportion of alcohols in them tends to be associated with flowers and to be a pleasant gentle smell such as rose or geranium.

Monoterpenols Monoterpenols are most commonly found in essential oils and include geraniol (in palmarosa), linalol (in lavender and neroli), terpineol-4 (in large quantities in tea tree oil) and citronellol (in rose and geranium). They are strong anti-infective agents, being antibacterial and antiviral. There are many reports on the use of essential oils against infections of various pathologies, but most of these have investigated the use of whole essential oils. It is difficult, therefore, to attribute their effectiveness specifically to monoterpenols, particularly as it may be the synergistic blend of a variety of constituents that affects the infective organisms. Mono-terpenols are also known to be stimulating and energizing, and to have low toxicity.

Sesquiterpenols Sesquiterpenols are formed when the hydroxyl group attaches to a sesquiterpene molecule; they are decongestant and generally toning to the body. A few sesquiterpenols are thought to act as cardiac or hepatic stimulants. An example of a sesquiter-penol is farnesol, found in frankincense.

Diterpenols Diterpenols, like diterpenes, are heavier than their mono- or sesqui- counterparts, making them less volatile, so they are less frequently found in essential oils. Chemically they are similar in structure to human steroids and consequently can help in balancing the endocrine system; an example is sclareol found in clary sage.

Aldehydes Aldehydes are formed when carbon atoms are joined by a hydrogen atom and a carboxyl group (carbon and oxygen linked by a double bond) but are not within a carbonic chain. However, the double bond means that aldehydes can break down relatively easily so will oxidize quickly, and this process is self-catalysing. As oxidation occurs, aldehydes are converted to acids which can be astringent and often act as a catalyst for other reactions.

It is important, therefore, to store and blend essential oils containing significant amounts of aldehydes with care. If an aromatherapist is considering adding essential oils to soaps, those that contain mainly alcohols rather than aldehydes should be selected as the latter will react with the alkaline nature of the soap to form salts such as sodium benzoate.

Aldehydes tend to smell quite sharp; for example, the aroma of almonds in sweet almond oil is due to the presence of benzyl aldehyde, which is also responsible for the rapid oxidation that can occur with this base oil. It is worth noting that approximately 1 per cent of the population is allergic to benzyl aldehyde, and that there is about 1–2 per cent benzyl aldehyde in sweet almond oil. This is a relatively small amount but it would be good practice to question clients about possible allergy to almonds if the therapist intends to use sweet almond as a carrier oil.

Some aldehydes are not terpenic, i.e. they are not made up of isoprene units, and, due to the presence of additional double bonds, are even more reactive than terpenic aldehydes, e.g. cinnamic aldehyde in cinnamon oil, which oxidizes readily to cinnamic acid.

Many of the aldehydes are skin irritants or sensitizers, so care should be taken when administering any oil with a high aldehyde proportion. This is especially so in the case of citral, which is found in bergamot, melissa and the citrus oils. The effects are worse, however, when the aldehyde is isolated from the whole essential oil. Aldehydes also have a sedative action and are generally calming, acting as a nerve tonic and reducing blood pressure and temperature. Certain aldehydes possess strong antiseptic properties, being antifungal, antiviral and antibacterial. In addition they can be used as anti-inflammatory agents.

Aldehydes are easily recognized as all the names end either in 'aldehyde' or in 'al', as in citronellal, geranial and neral.

Esters   When an acid and an alcohol combine, esters, together with water are formed; some are terpenoid, others non-terpenoid. They tend to have fruity pleasant aromas, and their names usually have the suffix 'ate', e.g. linalyl acetate found in clary sage oil. They have a mild action, are anti-inflammatory, calming and sedative, have a balancing action, and seem to possess antispasmodic properties.

The chemical reaction involving water is important in aromatherapy for, if water is added to an essential oil high in esters to produce a spray (for example to camomile oil which contains about 60 per cent esters), catalysis could occur which would reduce the amount and therefore the effects of the esters, but increase the proportion of acids and/or alcohols in the blend. It is thus recommended that any product involving water and ester-rich essential oils is used immediately and then discarded.

Ketones   A carboxyl group (oxygen plus carbon with a double bond) within a carbonic chain results in a ketone being formed. Ketones normally have the letters 'one' at the end of the name (camphor is an exception) and may be terpenic or non-terpenic.

Ketones have a valuable role to play in therapy for respiratory tract infections as they are expectorant and mucolytic, and are also cytophylactic. However, oils containing ketones should be used with care for some, such as thujone, found particularly in sage, thuja and pennyroyal oils, are known to be abortifacient if used to excess. Others can be neurotoxic when ingested, occasionally leading to epileptic fits, as in the case of pinocamphone in essential oil of hyssop. When using essential oils that contain ketones, it is wise to blend them in very low dilutions and avoid prolonged administration; in midwifery, ketone-containing oils are contraindicated during pregnancy until more research evidence is available to demonstrate their safety.

Phenols   Phenols are formed when an alcohol hydroxyl group attaches itself to a benzene ring. Electronically, phenols are uniformly stable and strongly positive, which makes them chemically very active. Many of the names end in 'ol' which can cause confusion with alcohols, but some end in 'ole' such as fenchole in fennel oil.

Phenols are well known as strong antiseptic and antibacterial agents, and as stimulants of the immune and nervous systems. However, they are also skin irritants so they should be blended in low dilutions.

Oxides   1.8 Cineole, sometimes known as eucalyptol(e), is the most commonly occurring oxide in essential oils. Chemically oxides are formed when the oxygen in a ring structure links two carbon molecules. Oxides share similarities with phenols, and should therefore be treated with the same caution in respect of skin irritation. 1.8 Cineole is a strong expectorant, mucolytic and decongestant; it is found in eucalyptus and thyme oils in large amounts and as a trace in many other oils.

Coumarins   Coumarins, a type of lactone, are what gives new-mown grass its characteristic smell. They are not volatile substances and therefore are found only in essential oils obtained by solvent extraction or expression—primarily the citrus essences—rather than those extracted by steam distillation.

Furocoumarins   Furocoumarins are photosensitizers and cause the development of irregular pigmentation and potential burning if skin is exposed to the sun directly after using oils containing them. These include bergapten found in bergamot oil.

Chapter 4

Effects of Essential Oils on the Body

Pharmacokinetics Aromatherapy is often derided by sceptics as a 'hobby' that employs pleasantly smelling oils to relax people by applying them through massage. The truth, of course, is very different. The chemical constituents are responsible for various therapeutic effects of essential oils, but these constituents also make them toxic if misused or abused.

To improve the status, respectability and credibility of aromatherapy it is vital that practitioners are aware of the potential dangers of some of the essential oils, especially when demonstrated through research, and take steps to utilize the oils safely and effectively. It is no longer sufficient for practitioners to recount anecdotal experiences without scientific backup, nor should they use oils with which they are unfamiliar. A code of practice for aromatherapists should be devised in which, amongst other things, it should be specified that practitioners should not use certain controversial essential oils without adequate preparation, in much the same way that nurses, midwives and health visitors are bound by their codes of practice (UKCC, 1992c, 1994), *Standards for the Administration of Medicines* (UKCC, 1992b) and *The Scope of Professional Practice* (UKCC, 1992a).

This requires an understanding not only of the chemical constituents but also of the pharmacokinetics of aromatherapy, as well as exploration of the possible side-effects and adverse reactions of aromatherapy oils. At present there is no centralized system for the reporting of potential reactions, as is the case with the 'yellow card' system for doctors to report complications from pharmaceutical preparations, although this is slowly changing (see p. 9).

Research into how and why essential oils work is limited, although increasing. There are several theories on the subject which merit further investigation. For example, the relaxation effects attributed to many essential oils may be due to their chemical properties or to the method of administration, particularly massage, or to a combination of the two factors. Alternatively the effects of oils may arise from the preference of the recipient for a certain type of smell which they either like and which makes them feel good, or dislike and may feel depressed by. On the other hand, these oils may be working directly on the central nervous system and so have an effect on the client's mood. Another theory is that essential oils in some way possess their own energies which interact with the human body's innate healing capabilities. This supposition would be extremely difficult to research and is one which professionals in conventional health care may find hard to understand or believe.

The body metabolizes essential oils via the normal pathways, in the same way that drugs are dealt with. Essential oils are fat soluble and are absorbed via cell membranes which are rich in lipids. It is possible that they may regulate immune function by lodging in the membrane of leucocytes, or affect nerve function as do anaesthetic drugs (Balacs, 1991a). The actions of essential oils may also be enhanced when administered via massage, which stimulates the circulation; damaged or diseased epidermis increases the rate of absorption into the bloodstream. It must be remembered, too, that some molecules of the essential oil are inhaled during the massage.

Essential oils are absorbed readily into the central nervous system for the brain is lipid rich, and into the liver via the bloodstream. They pass more slowly into muscle fibres, and finally into adipose tissue with its low blood flow. However, because adipose tissue acts as a reservoir for fat-soluble molecules, essential oils that reach fat tissue are probably stored there for some time. It is for this reason that clients are normally told not to bathe for several hours after an aromatherapy massage to allow the essential oils to take their full effect. On the other hand, it is necessary to investigate whether any changes occur to essential oil molecules while they are retained in the adipose tissue and, if so, whether the altered chemicals could have adverse effects on the client.

Essential oils, especially those containing ketones, esters and aldehydes, are thought to bind with plasma albumin. This will initially reduce the effects of the oil as the plasma albumin 'mops up' the oil molecules, but will also prolong the amount of time the essential oil remains in the body. In clients with low plasma albumin levels, such as those with impaired renal function, it would be wise to use much lower doses than normal to avoid the risk of high circulating levels of essential oil components (Balacs, 1992c).

Medical practitioners, understandably, are also concerned about the interactions between essential oils and drugs. It is obvious that where a client is receiving medication, for example to treat insomnia, an essential oil that is stimulating could potentially reverse the action of the drug. What is not known is whether the essential oil works via the same pathways as the drugs, or whether the effect is due to some other means of metabolism.

One trial conducted in 1969 by Jori and co-workers showed that certain essential oil components decreased the effects of pentabarbitol when tested in rats, which may have been due to an increase in liver enzyme activity caused by the essential oils. This would seem to indicate that the essential oils did not act directly on the same cells as the pentabarbitol, but rather exacerbated the excretion of the drug by speeding up detoxification in the liver.

The problem of dose-related effects also comes into question here. Jori and colleagues (1969) noted increased effects with higher doses, and this was also shown by Kovar *et al.* (1987) in their research into locomotor activity in mice following administration of rosemary oil. While the issue of dosages in aromatherapy requires further investigation, it is important for practitioners to acknowledge the relationship between the dose and the body-weight of the recipient, and to err on the side of caution. Lower doses should be used in small adults and, of course, in infants and children. Pregnant women are generally given lower proportions because of the risks of teratogenicity (see Chapter 5).

It is also important to understand the mechanism of both essential oils and prescribed drugs for, if the two substances compete to bind with plasma albumin, it is possible that the drug molecules will be left freely circulating in the blood. This could potentiate the action of the drug and lead to posssible overdose and/or adverse effects.

As with drugs, the chemicals in essential oils need to be metabolized and detoxified to aid absorption and excretion. Essential oil molecules are initially altered by oxidation, reduction or hydrolysis, mainly in the liver, but also partly by the lungs, intestinal mucosa, skin and plasma, depending on the route of administration.

The molecules are then conjugated before excretion. It is

interesting to note that one of the components of cinnamon oil has been found to reduce the level of hepatic glutathione, which is necessary for the conjugation of toxic substances, especially paracetamol (Boyland and Chasseau, 1970). For this reason cinnamon oil is contraindicated in clients taking paracetamol; conversely, clients who have received cinnamon oil as part of their aromatherapy treatment should be advised against taking paracetamol for the next 24 hours.

Essential oils are excreted in the main by the kidneys, although some constituents are expelled by means of expiration, and some such as citral, found in citrus fruit, are utilized via the cells as energy. Alcohols and aldehydes, which are comprised of small molecules, are excreted faster than terpenes, which are much larger molecules; molecules that bind to plasma albumin will be excreted more slowly. This may have implications for the use of essential oils in pregnancy when renal filtration is altered and larger molecules are filtered through into the urine more readily than normal.

Anatomy and physiology: where essential oils work

It is important to have a thorough working knowledge of the related anatomy and physiology in aromatherapy, and while there are many excellent textbooks available to which readers can refer, the subject is revisited here for midwives, for the sake of completeness. The systems covered are the physiology of olfaction; skin and the sense of touch; and the respiratory tract and respiration. As this book is aimed primarily at midwives, the anatomy of the female reproductive tract and the physiology of pregnancy, labour and the puerperium have not been included: it is assumed that readers will already be sufficiently familiar with it. However, readers who are aromatherapists without a midwifery qualification are strongly advised to review the subject and are referred to the list of recommended reading.

The physiology of olfaction   The sense of smell is extremely sensitive in human beings, although it is far from perfect. It is possible to detect over 100,000 odours, some in concentrations of up to one in 30 billion (Carola et al., 1992, p. 472), although some odours such as certain noxious gases cannot be detected.

Olfaction is classified as one of the special senses, with odour perception being transmitted directly to the brain via the first cranial nerve. High in the nasal cavity is the olfactory epithelium which contains the olfactory receptors or neurons, with a life of about 30 days; the supporting or sustentacular cells; and the basal cells, which divide to replace degenerating receptor and supporting cells.

For an aroma to be detected, the molecules of the substance must be volatile; in aromatherapy, volatile essential oil molecules pervade the air and some enter the nostrils and are picked up by the cilia at the vesicular end of the olfactory receptors. The cilia are surrounded by fluid secreted from the supporting cells and the olfactory (Bowman's) glands, in which the aromatic molecules dissolve prior to stimulation of the receptor sites. The research of Kobal *et al.* (1992) found that aromas were processed differently according to which nostril the molecules entered, a fact that may be due to pleasant and unpleasant smells being processed by different hemispheres of the brain. This would seem to be borne out by the research of Lorig *et al.* (1993) in which olfaction 'labelling' appears to be attributed to the left frontal brain.

The 'message' of the aroma is transmitted along the axons of the receptor cells to join other axons as part of the olfactory nerve, the fibres of which pass through the cribriform plate of the ethmoid bone in the roof of the nose to reach the olfactory bulb in the cerebrum. The olfactory bulb is actually an appendage of the brain and the axons of the neurons synapse with dendrites of other cells to form the olfactory glomeruli. The olfactory impulses are sorted in the glomeruli and pass into the olfactory tract, which passes directly to the primary cortex in the cerebrum (Fig. 4.1). Recent research collaboration between Germany and the UK has shown a possible trigeminal nerve involvement as well as the olfactory nerve activity (Kobal *et al.*, 1992).

Much work is being done on the effects of essential oil odours on the brain, and psychoaromatherapy is a growing field. Worwood (1990, p. 82) suggests that some essential oils stimulate the logical right side of the brain, while others stimulate the left side, a theory that is gaining credibility. When one considers the effects of the chemical components in pharmaceutical drugs, it is hardly surprising that those in essential oils should have physiologically induced effects on the psyche.

Japanese research found that machine operators' efficiency improved by 21 per cent when the atmosphere was scented with lavender, by 33 per cent when jasmine was used and by 54 per cent with lemon; subsequently an environmental fragrancing system has been developed to help increase productivity (Kallan, 1991).

The effects of odours on mood, creativity and perceived health have also been investigated (Knasko, 1992). This work showed that mood can be adversely affected by unpleasant odours with a

Fig 4.1 (a) Diagram
showing the olfactory
receptors and passage
of odours to the
olfactory bulb.
(b) Relationship of
olfactory bulb and
nerves to nose, palate
and brain.

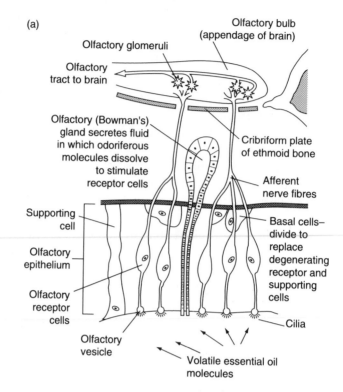

(a)

Olfactory bulb
(appendage of brain)

Olfactory glomeruli

Olfactory
tract to brain

Olfactory (Bowman's)
gland secretes fluid
in which odoriferous
molecules dissolve
to stimulate
receptor cells

Cribriform plate
of ethmoid bone

Afferent
nerve fibres

Supporting
cell

Basal cells–
divide to
replace
degenerating
receptor and
supporting
cells

Olfactory
epithelium

Olfactory
receptor
cells

Cilia

Olfactory
vesicle

Volatile essential oil
molecules

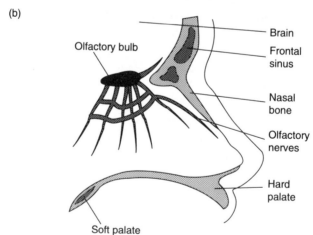

(b)

Brain

Olfactory bulb

Frontal
sinus

Nasal
bone

Olfactory
nerves

Hard
palate

Soft palate

corresponding effect on performance, and that fresh clean smells such as lemon result in perceptions of better health.

Slow brain waves, known as contingent negative variation, measured by electroencephalography, have been assessed to identify whether a selection of essential oils have the sedative or stimulant properties presumed by aromatherapists (Manley, 1993). The oils achieved the expected responses and included basil, bergamot, camomile, geranium, lemon, marjoram, neroli, patchouli, peppermint, rose, rosewood and sandalwood.

Similarly, locomotor activity of the brains of mice was shown to increase after administration of rosemary oil (Kovar *et al.*, 1987), and physiological responses to peppermint oil during sleep demonstrated significant differences between odour and non-odour periods, leading the researchers to postulate that 'relaxing' aromas may enhance sleep (Badia *et al.*, 1990). Neurodepressive effects were observed in mice and rats given two varieties of Spanish mint (Perez Raya *et al.*, 1990) and in mice who received oral *Lavandula augustifolia* oil (Guillemain *et al.*, 1989). The sedative effects of lavender oil have also been demonstrated by Buchbauer *et al.* (1991) and by Imberger and co-workers (1993), together with the excitory action of jasmine (Karamat *et al.*, 1992), although large doses of jasmine in mice have shown it to be a central nervous system depressant (Elisha *et al.*, 1988). Camomile, which is known to be sedative, has been shown to alter negative mood ratings to more positive ratings, inducing a degree of euphoria (Roberts and Williams, 1992).

In a holistic therapy such as aromatherapy it is impossible to separate the entities of body, mind and spirit, a concept that is only slowly being accepted by practitioners of conventional medicine. Psychoaromatherapy appears, however, to conform to biochemical principles and deserves much more investigation. What is, for some, even more difficult to understand is the notion that both the human body and essential oils, together with other organic substances, possess subtle energies that are capable of interacting. In a textbook aimed at exploring contemporary knowledge in relation to the use of essential oils for childbearing women, it is not feasible to discuss in depth the concept of potential subtle energies that may exist, for this is a relatively newly recognized area in Western clinical aromatherapy (although its origins are ancient), and readers are referred to the bibliography for further information.

Anatomy of the skin and the physiology of touch The skin is the largest organ in the body, occupying over 2 square metres, and is part of the integumentary system. Some areas of the body are covered with very thick skin, such as the middle of the back, while other parts, for example the eyelids, have a very thin covering. Skin acts as a protective cover for the internal organs, and prevents body fluids from being lost and harmful substances such as micro-organisms from gaining entry. It is virtually waterproof, but allows the passage of certain molecules, including therapeutic essential oils as well as harmful chemicals. When the body is warm, temperature control is achieved by means of the excretion of sweat, which cools on exposure to air, as well as by vasodilation and heat radiation; on cold days vasoconstriction in the skin acts as an insulating mechanism to retain body heat. Excretion of some waste materials such as urea and nitrogen occurs via the skin; and useful ultraviolet rays convert 7-dehydrocholesterol into vitamin D, whilst harmful ultraviolet light is screened out by the skin. Finally, the skin is an important sensory organ (see below).

The outer layer of skin, the epidermis, has no blood vessels but, as it is very thin, most cuts and abrasions penetrate the dermal layer beneath and so draw blood. Within the epidermis there are between three and five layers, depending on the thickness of the skin, starting with the stratum corneum and ending with the stratum spinosum and stratum basale, these latter two being cumulatively known as the stratum germinativum as they generate new cells. In addition, the palms of the hands and the soles of the feet contain the stratum lucidum and the stratum granulosum.

The stratum corneum consists of parallel rows of dead cells of soft keratin to maintain the skin's elasticity and to protect the living cells beneath from drying out due to exposure to the air. The dead cells are constantly being shed and replaced by cells pushed up from the germinative layer below. The palms and soles have the stratum lucidum next, which is also made up of dead cells and acts as an ultraviolet light filter to prevent sunburning of the areas. The stratum granulosum beneath the stratum lucidum contains granules of keratohyaline, which is needed for the process of keratinization or cell death. The stratum spinosum serves as a support and binding, and facilitates the process of protein synthesis leading to cell division and growth. The stratum basale divides the epidermis from the dermis and also helps to produce new cells to replace those lost at the surface.

The dermis or 'true' skin is a strong connective mesh of thick protein collagen fibres to make the skin tough, thinner but strong supporting reticular fibres, and elastic fibres for flexibility. The dermis also contains blood vessels, which carry the fat-soluble essential oil molecules around the body, lymphatic vessels, nerve fibres, glands and hair follicles, and is indefinably divided into a papillary and a reticular layer.

The papillary layer of loose connective tissue with bundles of collagenous fibres has tiny finger-like papillae which join it to the epidermal ridges. The papillae contain capillaries to nourish the epidermis as well as the special touch receptors called Meissner's corpuscles. The reticular layer of dense connective tissue has a mesh of collagenous fibre bundles forming a strong elastic network with a dominant directional pattern in different areas of the body. Tension lines in the skin resulting from the directional pattern of the fibres are called Langer's or cleavage lines; surgical incisions made parallel to the cleavage lines lead to more rapid healing and less scarring. Overstretching of the dermis during pregnancy can lead to tearing of the collagen and elastic fibres, with the repairing scar tissue resulting in striae gravidarum. Also within the reticular layer are blood and lymphatic vessels, nerves and free nerve endings, fat cells, sebaceous glands and hair roots. Pacinian corpuscles, or deep pressure receptors, are also found within this layer and in the subcuticular hypodermal layer. Muscle fibres are present as well in the reticular layer of the genital area and nipples.

The subcutaneous hypodermis of loose fibrous connective tissue is thick and has a rich supply of blood vessels, lymphatics and nerves as well as the bases of the hair follicles and sweat glands. In some parts of the body such as the breasts there are also thick layers of adipose cells (Fig. 4.2).

Sensory reception of the skin   A variety of sensations are perceived by the skin owing to the presence of sensory receptors, and in fact the sense of touch, once thought to be one sense, is actually a response to three stimuli: pressure, temperature and pain. Light touch without deformity of the skin surface is detected in the dermis by the free nerve endings and Meissner's corpuscles and in the epidermis of the palms and soles by free nerve endings and Merkel's corpuscles. Deep pressure results in the skin surface being temporarily deformed and is detected by Pacinian corpuscles or mechanoreceptors which measure pressure changes, situated in the dermis and subcutaneous layer of the skin. Variable vibrations of the skin are detected by Pacinian corpuscles, Meissner's corpuscles and corpuscles of Ruffini, depending on the frequency of vibration. Naked nerve endings can measure heat and cold, while specialized free nerve endings throughout the body are receptive to different

Fig 4.2 Diagram showing sensory receptors in the skin.

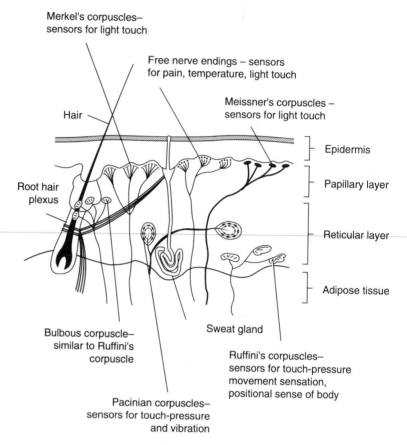

Merkel's corpuscles– sensors for light touch

Free nerve endings – sensors for pain, temperature, light touch

Meissner's corpuscles – sensors for light touch

Hair

Root hair plexus

Epidermis

Papillary layer

Reticular layer

Adipose tissue

Bulbous corpuscle– similar to Ruffini's corpuscle

Sweat gland

Ruffini's corpuscles– sensors for touch-pressure movement sensation, positional sense of body

Pacinian corpuscles– sensors for touch-pressure and vibration

types of pain. Continuous low-key stimulation of slow-conducting nerve fibres, mainly in the superficial layers of the skin, is thought to be the mechanism by which itches and ticklish sensations are perceived. The sensory neural pathways to the brain for both light touch and pain are situated in the spinothalamic tract ending in the cerebral cortex, and it is for this reason that effleurage (light massage) can act as a means of easing pain.

Aromatherapists constantly debate the issue of whether essential oils work because of their chemical constituents or because of the method of administration, especially massage. There is an increasing amount of research into this area and into the ability of essential oil molecules to be absorbed by the skin. Jager's and co-workers' (1992) trial using lavender oil in a massage showed constituents of the oil in the blood only 5 minutes after administration; they reached a peak at 20 minutes and were removed from the blood by 90 minutes. Weyers and Brodbeck (1989) tested the amounts of 1.8 cineole in skeletal muscle following dermal application of eucalyptus and found significant differences according to the method of application. There was a 320 per cent greater bioavailability of 1.8 cineole when an applicator was used compared with an occlusive dressing.

Massage is thought to increase the rate of systemic absorption of essential oils due to the increased blood flow. However, whilst it might be expected that a warm room, warm client and warm hands of the aromatherapist could increase absorption of the oils, it is probable that the molecules are more readily vaporized and are thus inhaled to take effect in the body. The most permeable areas of the skin for the passage of essential oil molecules are the palms of the hands and the soles of the feet, the forehead, scalp, axillae and, probably impractically, the scrotum. The legs, abdomen and trunk are less permeable but hirsute areas of the body facilitate the passage of molecules as they travel along the hair shaft to the dermal layer. Mucous membranes are highly permeable and essential oils should not be applied to these areas except in extremely low dilutions, as the area may become severely irritated.

The carrier oil used will also affect the rate of absorption, with many of the thicker more viscous carriers impairing the rate, although those rich in polyunsaturates will be absorbed fairly quickly. However, volatility of the essential oil molecules may be decreased by a particular carrier, thereby affecting the absorption rate, or skin enzymes may begin the process of metabolism of the molecules as happens with certain esters, notably benzyl acetate (Balacs, 1992b). Nevertheless, a group of skin enzymes called P450s which help to detoxify poisons, making them more water soluble prior to urinary excretion, may chemically alter some essential oils, in some cases producing toxins. This is known to be the case with pennyroyal, an essential oil completely contraindicated in aromatherapy, and may be responsible for the toxicity of other essential oils. This effect is significant for clients taking certain medications, for example lipid-lowering agents, steroids and anti-epileptic drugs such as phenobarbitone, in whom the drug's increased P450 activity could increase essential oil metabolism (Balacs, 1992b).

Physiology of respiration Inhalation of essential oil molecules plays a part in every aromatherapy treatment. Even when the method of administration is via the skin, some of the molecules will pervade the air and a few will enter the nostrils, passing directly to the brain to be perceived as an aroma, and affecting cerebral processes such as mood. Molecules also travel into the nasopharynx, the trachea and thence to the lungs, via the bronchi.

Within the lungs the bronchi divide further and further into a 'respiratory tree' and finally into respiratory bronchioles ending in the microscopic air sacs or alveoli, in which gaseous exchange occurs. Each lung contains over 350 million alveoli bunched in grape-like clusters, surrounded by capillaries. The alveolar and capillary walls are extremely thin to allow for the diffusion of oxygen and carbon dioxide between them. Once in the blood vessels oxygen and any other molecules carried with it are transported partially in solution and partially with haemoglobin around the body to be used as required.

It is obvious that, for some conditions involving the cardiorespiratory system, administration of essential oils by inhalation will be the treatment of choice, although Ryman (1991, p. viii) states this as her preferred route for almost all clients. It is also possible that certain components of the oils possess a particular affinity for specific organs in the body. Falk–Filipsson (1993), for example, suggests that monoterpenes are very soluble in blood, have a high respiratory uptake and are easily stored in adipose tissues, and showed an approximately 70 per cent pulmonary uptake of *d*–limonene after inhalation.

The absorption of essential oil molecules through inhalation and the effect of the fragrances on cerebral activity is not dependent on aroma perception. This has been shown by the work of Nasel *et al.* (1994) in which inhalation of 1.8 cineole by nine subjects (including one anosmic person) demonstrated similar effects on the general cerebral blood flow of all nine subjects. The authors postulated that inhalation of essential oils may have a direct pharmacological action on the brain, a fact that is increasingly being used to increase work efficiency and productivity (Sugano and Sato, 1991). This is further borne out by the increased attention span, concentration and efficiency that occurred irrespective of personal like or dislike of aromas, in the early work of Tasev *et al.* (1969), although Kikuchi and colleagues (1989) found that aroma preference did improve performance. Other work on human reaction times after inhalation of various essential oils has also been carried out (Sugano, 1989; Miyake *et al.*, 1991; Miyazaki *et al.*, 1991; Karamat *et al.*, 1992).

Chapter 5

Safety of Essential Oils in Pregnancy and Childbirth

The issue of safety of essential oils concerns all aromatherapists, but the specific problem of identifying which oils are safe to use in childbearing women is one that is still very much open to question. It is necessary first to consider general safety data available on essential oils and then to apply the principles to pregnancy, childbirth, lactation and the neonate.

Certain essential oils are completely contraindicated in aromatherapy because of their toxicity (Table 5.1). Others have uses only in perfumery rather than therapeutic aromatherapy. The main factors that govern the use of an essential oil for therapeutic use are phototoxicity, dermal and oral toxicity, carcinogenicity and general pharmacological effects. For midwives the issues centre around teratogenicity, mutagenicity, oils that are emmenagogic or abortifacient,

Table 5.1
Hazardous essential oils contraindicated in aromatherapy

Armoise (mugwort)   Arnica   Basil (exotic)   Birch (sweet)
Bitter almond   Boldo leaf   Broom   Buchu
Calamus   Camphor (brown or yellow)   Cassia   Chervil
Cinnamon bark   Clove (bud, leaf or stem)   Costus   Deertongue
Elecampane   Fennel (bitter)   Horseradish   Jaborandi leaf
Melilotus   Mustard   Origanum   Pennyroyal   Pine (dwarf)
Rue   Sassafras   Savin   Savory (summer)   Tansy   Thuja
Tonka   Vanilla   Wintergreen   Wormwood

and an understanding of how the physiology of pregnancy and the pharmacology of essential oils interact.

Midwives attempting to elicit information about safety of essential oils in pregnancy will find a plethora of conflicting and confusing advice, notably in books aimed at the consumer. Indeed, some readily available books for pregnant women contain misleading and occasionally potentially dangerous information. One of the main aromatherapy texts on safety (International School of Aromatherapy, 1993) suggests, correctly, that many other substances may adversely affect the fetus, for example alcohol, but fails to take into account the amount of research supporting this fact. In aromatherapy there is virtually no research into the effects on the fetus of essential oils administered to the mother during pregnancy. What little work has been carried out on expectant women *assumes* a degree of safety of the oils being used, merely through lack of evidence to the contrary. It is therefore vital that midwives using aromatherapy in their work err on the side of caution until more data are available.

Photoxicity

Certain essential oils are known to possess some phototoxic effects but the degree of the reaction is unknown in many oils. The information that is available has resulted from extensive testing of animals, but it is recognized that there are differences between the physiologies of the various animals tested and humans. Consequently the information can only be considered a guide until further research has been carried out. Of significance to midwives are the potential effects on the skin of essential oils known to cause photosensitivity at a time when there are raised melanocytic hormone levels circulating in the body. The citrus oils are generally quoted as having some degree of phototoxicity, which is of relevance in midwifery for these are otherwise considered to be the safest oils to use during pregnancy. Research in 1985 by Naganuma *et al.* demonstrated the active phototoxic ingredients of lemon oil samples from around the world to be mainly bergapten and partially oxypeucedanin, with the latter component also being found in samples of lime and bitter orange essence.

Essential oils considered to be phototoxic include bergamot, lemon, lime, mandarin, neroli, bitter and sweet orange, and possibly ginger. For practical purposes, women should be advised against direct exposure of the skin to the sun following administration of any of these oils, although it is likely that absorption into the body is completed rapidly, probably within 2 hours.

Dermal toxicity   Irritation of the skin has been reported on many occasions in relation to several different essential oils (Table 5.2), although this does seem to be dose related. Allergy to camomile oil has been recorded (Van Ketel, 1982; McGeorge and Steele, 1991), and a case of chemical burns resulting from contact with neat peppermint oil was reported by Parys (1983). Allergy to both dermal and oral application of tea tree oil was found to be due to the presence of eucalyptol (De Groot and Weyland, 1992), which may also be the cause of similar irritation to eucalyptus oil (Spoerke *et al.*, 1989), while benzoin has long been known to cause allergic reactions in sensitive individuals (Mann, 1982; Rademaker and Kirby, 1987; Tripathi *et al.*, 1990).

The issue of whether the aromatherapist could develop dermatitis from frequent use of different oils is important, and a trial is currently under way to investigate this (Wong, 1994). Certainly there are anecdotal reports from therapists about the effects on their hands; this author experiences itching after using camomile and a colleague is unable to use lavender oil for the same reason. Occupational allergy to lavender oil has also been reported in a hairdresser (Brandao, 1986); French marigold (tagetes) has resulted in eczematous rashes in one practitioner (Bilsland and Strong, 1990); and prolonged exposure to peppermint oil, an ingredient in several dental preparations, caused hypersensitivity in a dental technician (Dooms-Goossens *et al.*, 1977).

On some occasions the allergy may be due to a single chemical component of an oil, but as that component may be present in many different oils in varying proportions it is necessary to elicit the precise chemical cause. An example of this would be geraniol, a common constituent of several oils, but which has been shown to lead to

Table 5.2
Essential oils that may cause adverse skin reactions

Basil, French	Benzoin	Bergamot	Cedarwood, Virginian
Camomile, German, Roman		Cinnamon (leaf)	Citronella
Geranium (especially Bourbon)		Ginger (in high concentrations)	
Jasmine?	Lavender	Lemon	Lemongrass	Melissa
Peppermint	Orange, sweet?	Tea tree	Thyme

dermatitis (Guerra *et al.*, 1987). Cinnamon leaf may also cause irritation (Calnan, 1976).

There are accounts of skin complaints arising from the extended use of an essential oil or a substance containing an essential oil, (Sharma *et al.*, 1987), but this should not be a problem for clients receiving professional aromatherapy as it is generally believed that no single oil should be used continuously for more than 3 weeks.

The quality of an essential oil should be taken into account when considering the possibility of dermal toxicity, for the pure organic oils should not be contaminated. Oxidation and ageing may also trigger skin reactions, so it is wise to discard oils that are past their recommended shelf-life. Research in 1969 by Woeber and Krombach supported the use of pure, good quality, non-oxidized oils and suggested that the substances produced in the extraction process of some low-grade essential oils could act as skin sensitizers. Rudski and colleagues (1976) investigated sensitivity to 35 essential oils and found that, as well as those expected to cause reactions such as bitter orange, bergamot, geranium and eucalyptus, others including ylang ylang, cedarwood and citronella gave positive results.

Experiments on rabbits have led to the production of monographs by the Research Institute of Fragrance Materials (RIFM) which are used by the perfumery and food industries and by aromatherapists. Nevertheless the RIFM recognizes the need for additional research as there are different rates of skin absorption between rabbits and humans, and the monographs can therefore be used only as a guide.

Japanese research is cited in one of the safety guides available (International School of Aromatherapy, 1993, p. 12) in which a large-scale study of 200 volunteers over 8 years using well over a quarter of a million patch tests identified certain factors regarding skin sensitivity to essential oils. These included the facts that men were more sensitive than women and that sensitivity in many subjects was increased around the time of change of season. Of significance to midwives is the observation that illness and stressful situations—including pregnancy—resulted in a greater degree of skin sensitivity than normal.

Oral toxicity Essential oils are used by medically qualified aromatherapists in Europe, notably France, as an alternative or complement to conventional pharmaceutical preparations. Jean Valnet is the contemporary leading authority on the gastrointestinal administration of essential oils. Some aromatherapy books, including those for the consumer, advocate the use of small amounts of essential oils in cookery (e.g. Worwood, 1990). While it is perfectly probable that essential oils may be both pleasant and safe to use in this way, aromatherapists in the UK do not prescribe essential oils orally unless the practitioner is very experienced. It is not possible to monitor the rate of absorption via the intestinal mucosa, and insufficient is known about the changes that may occur to essential oils in the gut.

There are some reports of poisoning from the ingestion of large amounts of essential oils such as citronella (Temple *et al.*, 1991) and eucalyptus (Gurr and Scroggie, 1965; Spoerke *et al.*, 1989). Some therapeutic work has, however, been done with essential oils in capsule form, for example peppermint (Somerville *et al.*, 1984) and garlic (Joshi *et al.*, 1987). Controversy has arisen recently over the proposal by one eminent leader in British aromatherapy to offer a postbasic course in the internal uses of essential oils when it is generally felt that this method of administration should be used only by medically qualified doctors.

For pregnant women the culinary use of herbs enables them to receive the therapeutic effects of the plant without the concentration of essential oils administered in other ways; neither will it lead to potential gastric irritation or uncertain absorption rate of ingesting essential oils.

From a safety viewpoint it is vital that essential oils are stored out of reach of children and that any blends given to women for home use are labelled 'not for internal use'.

Carcinogenicity

Little information is available regarding the potential carcinogenic and cytotoxic effects of essential oils. Those oils recognized to have a strong carcinogenic possibility, including camphor, sassafras and calamus, are already contraindicated in aromatherapy (International School of Aromatherapy, 1993, pp. 93–95). The dangers of these essential oils are due to the high levels of safrole, but it would perhaps be wise to refrain from using any oil containing safrole in pregnancy; this includes cinnamon and nutmeg. Basil is also thought to have a potential carcinogenic effect if used in large doses (Anthony, 1987, and Zangouras *et al.*, 1981, both cited by Tisserand and Balacs, 1995, p. 120).

It would appear that more work is being carried out on the *anti-cancer* effects of essential oils than on the tumour-inducing effects (Fang *et al.*, 1989; de la Puerta *et al.*, 1993; Zheng *et al.*, 1993).

Teratogenicity and mutagenicity

Similarly, there is a dearth of data on possible effects on the fetus, perhaps due to the ethicolegal minefield involved in undertaking research on human subjects. Even the Aromatherapy Organizations Council, currently investigating the contemporary use of essential oils in human pregnancy rather than in animals, is working from the premise that aromatherapists might elicit information on the maternofetal effects of essential oils *assumed* to be safe at this time (Anonymous, 1994c). Personal communications of this author with both midwives and aromatherapists have highlighted an alarming plethora of oils being used on pregnant women. Some of these oils are, at the least, controversial and are often extremely dangerous.

By their very nature essential oils will cross the placental barrier and have the potential to affect the fetus. It is becoming a matter of urgency to investigate this in more depth as the number of pregnant women using essential oils increases.

High levels of sabinyl acetate in *Juniperus sabinus* and *Plecanthrus fruticosus* are thought to be the cause of abortion and fetal malformations in mice. However, Pages *et al.* (1990) tested *Eucalyptus globuli*, which also contains sabinyl acetate, on mice and found no toxic effects on embryos or fetuses, which suggests that toxicity is related to the proportion of the relevant constituent. Cinnamic aldehyde, present in large quantities in cinnamon bark and cassia oils, has also been shown to be teratogenic in animals (Mantovani *et al.*, 1989, cited by Balacs, 1992a) but, as can be seen in Table 5.1, these essential oils are contraindicated in aromatherapy in any case.

Abortifacient and emmenagogic essential oils

There is no evidence to suggest that essential oils classed as emmenagogic will also be abortifacient. However, it is probably wise, until more research has been carried out, to avoid emmenagogic oils (Table 5.3) in the first trimester of pregnancy, although a few of these may be used with caution in low dilution towards term for specific purposes, for example on the legs for oedema or via inhalation for sinus congestion. Tisserand and Balacs (1995, p. 110) argue that there is no justification for restricting essential oil use to certain specified periods during pregnancy, and that caution should be exercised throughout the antenatal phase with any oils which are potentially hazardous. It is also probably wise to limit the use of emmenagogic essential oils during the early puerperium when lochia are being discharged.

Most of the reports of fatal or near-fatal reactions to essential oils in pregnancy are related to those oils already contraindicated for

Table 5.3 Essential oils thought to be emmenagogic	Aniseed (narcotic, oestrogenic) Angelica Basil (?carcinogenic) Bay (narcotic) Calamintha (hallucinogenic) Caraway Carrot seed Cedarwood (abortifacient) Celery seed Calendula Camomile Cinnamon leaf (hepatotoxic) Citronella Clary sage Cumin Cypress Fennel (narcotic, oestrogenic) Frankincense Galbanum Hyssop (moderately toxic, hypertensive) Jasmine Juniper (abortifacient) Labdanum Lavender Marjoram Melissa Peppermint Myrrh (?toxic in large doses) Nutmeg Parsley (toxic in large doses) Rose Rosemary (hypertensive) Sage Tarragon (?carcinogenic) Thyme (?toxic in large doses)			

This list refers specifically to essential oils and does not preclude the culinary use of the herbs mentioned, in which the amount of essential oil would be minimal. In any case the emmenagogic action of an essential oil does not necessarily mean that it is contraindicated during pregnancy (see below).

therapeutic aromatherapy use. Pennyroyal, for example, is not used because of its pulegone content. Pulegone is a monoterpenic ketone which may cause serious hepatic disease or failure, so is not used for *any* client, let alone those compromised by the physiological upheaval of pregnancy. Balacs (1992a) recounts several obstetric incidents involving pennyroyal which have been reported in medical journals since the end of the nineteenth century. In some cases the women were unsuccessful in their attempts to induce abortion but suffered a variety of severe toxic effects, occasionally resulting in death.

The hepatic effects of pennyroyal have been found to be due to pulegone, isopulegone and menthofuran, although certain liver enzymes may help to metabolize pulegone to a less toxic level. When spontaneous abortion occurs with pennyroyal, or other toxic oils such as tansy or rue, it is probably as a result of maternal (rather than fetal) *poisoning*, and no proven abortifacient action can be attributed to these oils.

Research by Toaff *et al.* in 1979, in which mice were given regular doses of citral, did not elicit toxic effects but did demonstrate a reduction in the number of ovarian follicles, ovum implantations, litter size and, consequently, successful pregnancy outcome. The adverse effects were attributed to the high doses of citral but the authors also raised questions regarding prolonged administration of lower doses of citral-containing essential oils during human pregnancy. Although this research does not appear to have been replicated since the late 1970s, it does highlight potential issues of concern for the use of essential oils in pregnancy, particularly as those oils most frequently claimed to be relatively safe are the very oils that contain citral, such as grapefruit, lemon, lime, mandarin, orange, petitgrain and tangerine.

Essential oils with systemic effects undesirable in pregnancy

Midwives need to be aware of the effects of any essential oil which they use in their practice, for although some may be considered acceptable in pregnancy, in that they are not abortifacient or emmenagogic, they may cause other unwanted responses which can adversely affect either the mother or the fetus.

For example, some essential oils may cause hypertension or hypotension. Using a hypotensive oil for a woman with pregnancy-induced hypertension could have the desired therapeutic effect, but this same oil would not be selected for a labouring woman in whom epidural analgesia was causing a fall in blood pressure. Essential oils considered to be hypertensives are rosemary, sage, thyme, hyssop and camphor; these are also emmenagogic so should not be used in pregnancy, but rosemary is occasionally useful in labour. Oils which reduce blood pressure include clary sage, garlic, lavender, lemon, marjoram, melissa and ylang ylang. It is interesting to read that Tisserand and Balacs (1995, p. 65) do not consider essential oils to be contraindicated in cases of hypertension or hypotension, as there is insufficient evidence to suggest that they are hazardous. They list certain constituents as being hypotensors: linalol, citronellol, nerol, geraniol, terpineol and cineole (in descending order of effectiveness).

Certain oils are known to trigger epileptic fits and should be avoided in women with epilepsy and in those with fulminating pre-eclampsia (although as they are also hypertensive they would not be used in the latter group); these include sage, fennel, hyssop and rosemary.

Interactions with pharmaceutical drugs should also be considered, although those listed by Tisserand and Balacs (1995, p. 43) are generally essential oils not normally used for pregnancy and childbearing.

Nutmeg is contraindicated in mothers receiving pethidine, and care should be taken when using essential oils in conjunction with certain tranquillizers, anticonvulsants and antihistamines—although it is probably wise to check biosynthetic pathways and drug interactions for any woman before using essential oils. This will not usually pose a problem for midwives as most of the women for whom they care are fit and healthy and unlikely to be receiving medication; those already under medical supervision will possibly not be suitable for the administration of essential oils. Geranium is reputed to have an anticoagulant effect and is therefore contra-indicated in women receiving warfarin, although aromatherapy for these women and those with cardiac disease should be administered only after full consultation between the consultants and the midwife, who should be a fully trained and experienced therapist. It is worth noting, however, that some oils stimulate the heart and should be used with caution in all women during pregnancy and the puerperium when massive cardiovascular adaptations are taking place. These include black pepper, caraway, cinnamon, hyssop, nutmeg and thyme.

Rubefacient (warming) oils would be unsuitable for pyrexial women, as would those which increase perspiration. These include basil, black pepper, cajeput, camomile, eucalyptus, fennel, garlic, ginger, hyssop, juniper, lavender, melissa, myrrh, peppermint, rosemary and tea tree, although the latter is valuable in cases where the pyrexia is due to infection.

Most essential oils are excreted via the kidneys, but certain oils increase diuresis and can be helpful for retention or postpartum oedema. They are contraindicated, however, after severe blood loss. Essential oils in this category include benzoin, black pepper, carrot seed, cedarwood, camomile, cypress, eucalyptus, fennel, garlic, geranium, hyssop, juniper, lavender, lemon, parsley, patchouli, rose, rosemary, sage and sandalwood.

These examples demonstrate the importance of a thorough understanding of both the physiology of the childbearing phase and the potential effects of essential oils on either the mother or the fetus. Oils that can be used to treat specific conditions are discussed more fully in Part 2.

In labour the same criteria for selection of oils as in pregnancy should be considered, although some of those that are considered abortifacient can be used with care, but they would be contraindicated in women at risk of haemorrhage. Postnatally it is necessary to be aware of the history of pregnancy and labour, and then to review the desirable and unacceptable effects of the oils to be used. Obviously many essential oils that were contraindicated in pregnancy may now be used, although those that induce uterine bleeding should be administered with caution until the lochia have subsided. For the neonate only very low dilutions (i.e. 0.5–1 per cent) of gentle essential oils should be used, and it is advised that this is restricted to camomile or mandarin. In many instances simple massage with a base oil can be effective and is certainly safer if there is any doubt about individual essential oils. The fragility of the skin in preterm neonates does, however, mean that any massage should be performed extremely gently.

Conclusion

It is vital that the possible dangers of essential oils are recognized. The lack of adequate research findings in relation to pregnancy and childbearing means that both midwives and aromatherapists currently have limited knowledge on which to base their practice. Great caution should be exercised when caring for pregnant women who wish to receive aromatherapy. It is not the intention of the author to dissuade midwives completely from using essential oils in their practice, but rather to highlight the effects that the chemistry or pharmacological actions may have upon clients. Even those midwives who do not personally utilize essential oils should advise women to purchase only good-quality products and to use them in very low dilutions, preferably with reference to a qualified aromatherapist for the most appropriate blends.

This author would strongly advise midwives and aromatherapists treating pregnant women to use only the lowest doses necessary to achieve the desired results, avoiding prolonged administration of any one oil (or those with similar levels of the same constituents), and to refrain from using essential oils until the second trimester. Practitioners must be able to justify their choice of essential oils and must know thoroughly the actions, contraindications and side-effects of oils which they administer. While these principles apply to the use of aromatherapy for all clients, special attention must be paid to the fact that two human beings are being treated during pregnancy; and for midwives, their primary duty lies in working within the boundaries of the UK Central Council's regulations, in order to protect their clients.

PART 2

The Art of Aromatherapy in

Midwifery Practice

Chapter 6

Administration of Essential Oils

Essential oils can be administered in many ways: via the skin or mucous membranes through massage, baths, compresses or douches (Tisserand (1992, p. 82) suggests they may also be given as enemas), or via the respiratory tract as inhalations or in vaporizers. Essential oils may also be given orally to be absorbed through the gastro-intestinal tract, but should be prescribed only by very experienced or medically qualified aromatherapists; this route of administration is not considered here.

The choice of method may depend on several factors. First, the condition being treated may dictate the route of administration; for example, a cough or cold is best treated with inhalations so that the essential oils act directly on the respiratory tract. On the other hand, women seeking aromatherapy for the relief of stress would benefit most from a massage; many research trials are concerned with deciding whether the relaxation obtained is a result of the chemical constituents of the essential oils or of the massage itself (see Part 1).

Second, particularly within midwifery practice, factors such as time may play a part. This might lead to the decision to use essential oils in the bath or bidet rather than giving a massage which requires a longer period of undisturbed time than may be available. However, when more or less continuous one-to-one care is given, as in the delivery suite, massage can be appropriate for relieving pain and helping to relax the mother.

Third, and perhaps most importantly, the preference of the client for a particular method must be taken into account. Some women dislike being touched, especially during labour, and this must be respected by offering alternative ways of receiving essential oils; others prefer showering to bathing so that adding essential oils to the bathwater is not feasible.

Fourth, professional accountability of the midwife must be considered, including ethicolegal, health and safety, and educational issues (see Chapter 1).

Application through the skin: massage

The application of an essential oil blend via the skin is enhanced when given via massage, which in itself can be mentally and physically relaxing, yet revitalizing. Massage helps to stimulate circulatory and excretory processes (urinary, intestinal, lymphatic and integumentary), relaxes and tones muscles, and assists the individual quite literally to 'get in touch' with herself.

There are many types of massage, which are often used in conjunction with one another. The commonest types used in aromatherapy involve a combination of Swedish soft-tissue massage, deeper lymphatic and neuromuscular massage, shiatsu and reflexology. The specific system of therapeutic touch is actually a misnomer as it does not involve physical touching of the skin but instead concentrates on massaging the aura and is not dealt with in this book. Where the term 'therapeutic touch' is used, it refers simply to the therapeutic effects that physical touch (massage) can have on individuals.

In this book, with the emphasis on the use of essential oils, it is not the intention to teach the reader *how* to perform massage. Basic principles are discussed and some suggestions for the application of manual techniques to midwifery practice are made, but it is left to the practitioner to pursue the acquisition of specific skills elsewhere. Massage is, in any case, mostly intuitive; massage cannot be learnt from a book and there are many excellent courses (and more detailed course texts) available (see list of suggested further reading/useful addresses).

Swedish soft-tissue massage   Swedish massage consists of several types of movement: stroking (effleurage) kneading, percussion movements and deep thumb massage called petrissage.

Effleurage   Effleurage is a slow flowing movement in which the body is stroked by the whole hand, which changes shape to fit the contours of the body. Movements are normally directed towards the heart to stimulate circulation and lymphatic drainage, although effleurage at the end of a massage tends to be outwards from the limbs and upwards from the head in an attempt to remove tension from the body, and either to sedate or to stimulate the recipient. Effleurage may be fairly light for work on the nervous system and for helping to relax the woman emotionally, although not so light as to cause tickling sensations. It may also be a deeper movement for work on specific tense muscles and to improve blood flow.

Effleurage is used to link other movements and can be performed on any part of the body; if in doubt about what to do in a massage, effleurage will enhance a woman's sense of relaxation and wellbeing. The tendency of the novice masseuse to work too lightly will be overcome with increasing confidence, and practitioners will come to know the most appropriate pressure to use. For example, the back and limbs often respond to deep firm pressure, whereas the pregnant or labouring woman may want featherlight effleurage in a clockwise circular movement over the abdomen. She can be shown how to do this herself during pregnancy and many women report the calming of a very active fetus when they have done so. Similarly, effleurage of the face will need a much lighter touch, as will babies—in this latter case pressure will instinctively be adjusted by the midwife in much the same way as she adapts the pressure of cardiopulmonary resuscitation for adults or babies.

Effleurage can be performed with one hand or both, either together or alternatively; in straight flowing lines following the contours of the body or in circles of varying sizes. Different pressures and speeds, perhaps even pausing and holding occasionally, will provide variety in the massage and prevent boredom in both the recipient and the therapist.

Petrissage Petrissage involves deeper work with the thumbs on more precise areas of the body and may be effective in reducing motor neuron excitability (Morelli *et al.*, 1990; Sullivan *et al.*, 1991; Goldberg *et al.*, 1992). Soft tissues, primarily muscles, are compressed, either against underlying bone or against themselves, and the movements may be in the form of kneading, wringing, rolling or shaking manipulations.

Kneading Kneading is a circular, squeezing movement performed with the whole hand, using the fingers and thumbs to pick up fleshy parts of the body or to compress the tissues against the underlying structures. The movement may be performed with the whole hand, the palm, the fingers, or the tips of the fingers and thumbs.

Kneading is a very useful technique for dealing with aching, tense muscles as it stimulates the local circulation and disperses any lactic acid that may have built up in the muscles. Spontaneous massage of the shoulders is a kneading movement of the flesh over the trapezius muscle.

Occasionally the tissues of the body are compressed using a 'picking up' technique to lift, squeeze and release them. In a wringing movement, the tissues are compressed, lifted and then pulled and pushed by alternate hands, while another technique involves rolling the skin and, in some instances, the underlying muscles.

Percussion movements Percussion movements (sometimes called tapotement) include cupping and hacking, which are perhaps the two movements most readily associated with Swedish massage. They involve brisk, bouncy movements on fleshy parts of the body to improve circulation and to re-energize the recipient. Hacking is done with the distal edges of the hands which bounce alternately, at right angles to the client's body, and has been shown to improve blood flow in skeletal muscle (Hovind and Nielson, 1974).

Cupping movements are performed with the therapist's palms directed downwards and slightly arched; this is the action carried out by physiotherapists to stimulate chest drainage. Both cupping and hacking should be followed by effleurage to soothe and calm; in some cases these movements are omitted altogether as they may disturb the client's deep relaxation, particularly when the aim of massage is to induce sleep.

Benefits of massage Generally, massage has been found to reduce heart and respiratory rates and blood pressure (Barr and Taslitz, 1970) (Table 6.1 and 6.2), although concern for cardiothoracic patients led to a trial which did not demonstrate significant cardiovascular changes (Bauer and Dracup, 1987). Cardiovascular instability was put forward as a possible contraindication to massage in critically ill patients (Hill, 1993) (see Table 6.3 for contraindications). Massage does, however, increase the individual's sense of wellbeing (McKechnie et al., 1983; Sims, 1986; Farrow, 1990; Field et al., 1993; Fraser and Kerr, 1993) and reduce pain perception (Day et al., 1987; Ginsberg and Famaey, 1987; Kaada and Torsteinbo, 1989; Ferrell-Torry and Glick, 1993) (Table 6.1). Women who receive touch during labour, particularly in the transition phase, have been shown to be more relaxed, to have

Table 6.1
Benefits of massage

Physical	Psychological
Muscle relaxation	Mental relaxation
Sudorific	Revitalizing
Lowers blood pressure	Releases emotions
Stimulates circulation	Facilitates communication
Increases diuresis	Aids sleep
Stimulates lymphatic drainage	Time for oneself
Reduces oedema	
Pain relieving	

lower blood pressures, to experience less pain and to feel more satisfied post-delivery than control subjects who were not touched (Birch, 1986; Hedstrom and Newton, 1986; Le May, 1986). Perception of pain can be adversely or positively affected by a woman's mental state, so that fear and anxiety will exacerbate the

Table 6.2
Preparation for massage

Practitioner

Hand exercises to keep hands supple and comfortable
Remove watch, rings and other jewellery; wash hands
Time management—allow sufficient time for client
Wear comfortable clothes, but not so loose that they will hang around the client
Ensure own physical comfort—posture, empty bladder, etc.
'Tune in' to client—mentally and physically, e.g. breathing
Warm hands, pour oil into own hands not on to client
Learn to 'see' with the hands

Environment

Warm, ventilated, private and peaceful room
Consider lighting, music, visual impact of room, e.g. colour
Firm couch, correct height, covered with towels
Towels to cover client, support back, neck, etc.
Ensure no disturbances—telephone, etc.
Oils ready for blending; tissues available for spillages

Client

Ensure feeling of security and partnership
Physical comfort—warm, empty bladder
Take history from client; mutual decision regarding blend
Make comfortable on couch, well supported
Facilitate relaxation, breathing, etc.
Expose only the part of body being massaged
Be sensitive to verbal and non-verbal signs from client

Table 6.3
Contraindications and
precautions of massage

General
Infection, contagious disease, pyrexia
Skin problems—inflammation, open wounds, burns, severe bruising
Varicosities—avoid direct pressure
Thrombophlebitis or phlebothrombosis
Sciatica—take care around this area
Recent fractures, scars—avoid direct pressure
Carcinoma—avoid direct massage over relevant area
Recent immunizations—avoid direct pressure
Immediately after ingestion of heavy meal or alcohol
Hypotension—monitor blood pressure closely
Preference of client

Pregnancy: specific
Sacral and suprapubic massage during first trimester
Deep massage of calves if history of thrombosis
Brisk heel massage—reflexology zone for pelvic area
Shiatsu points contraindicated in pregnancy (see Fig. 6.1)
Hypotension or fainting episodes—monitor blood pressure closely
Abdominal massage if history of antepartum haemorrhage
Uncertainty of midwife—if in doubt, refrain
Preference of client

pain, while nurturing care will assist in reducing it. This may be due to the release of pituitary endorphins, which facilitate a sense of wellbeing; the transmission of pain impulses to the brain may be interrupted; and inhibitory interneurons in the spinal cord are stimulated to lessen the pain perception.

It is also possible that various blood changes may occur as a result of massage, including an increase in the levels of creatinine kinase, lactase dehydrogenase, growth hormone and adrenocorticotrophic hormone (Arkko et al., 1983) and a decrease in blood and plasma viscosity, haematocrit (Ernst et al., 1987) and, 24 hours after the massage, haemoglobin (Arkko et al., 1983).

Shiatsu   Shiatsu techniques are often incorporated into aromatherapy massage and are thought to rebalance energy along the meridians (energy flow lines) throughout the body. Although it was traditionally believed that meridians were metaphorical, recent work has demonstrated their physical existence as shown by electrical energy tests and radio-opaque dye tests (Bensoussan, 1991)

Expert shiatsu practitioners carry out full-body massage by work-

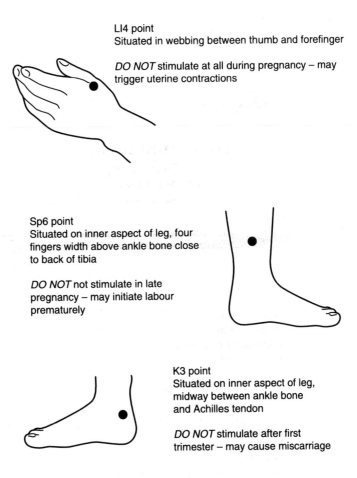

Fig 6.1 Shiatsu points contraindicated in pregnancy.

LI4 point
Situated in webbing between thumb and forefinger

DO NOT stimulate at all during pregnancy – may trigger uterine contractions

Sp6 point
Situated on inner aspect of leg, four fingers width above ankle bone close to back of tibia

DO NOT not stimulate in late pregnancy – may initiate labour prematurely

K3 point
Situated on inner aspect of leg, midway between ankle bone and Achilles tendon

DO NOT stimulate after first trimester – may cause miscarriage

ing along each meridian of the body, but in aromatherapy only a few points are used. It is perfectly feasible for midwives to learn sufficient techniques to apply shiatsu to their practice and to be able to use them safely. There are certain shiatsu points that should not be stimulated during pregnancy as they may initiate preterm labour (Fig. 6.1). It is also important to ensure that the techniques are learnt properly to avoid any potential complications. *The Lancet* of February 1993 carried a report of a woman who developed herpes zoster lesions 3 days after receiving what appeared to be an over-vigorous shiatsu massage. The authors surmise that nerve root damage may have occurred either during the massage or as a result of tissue inflammation (Mumm *et al.*, 1993).

Finger pressure is applied slowly and rhythmically, never abruptly or forcefully. This slow work enables the tissues and organs of the body to respond to the treatment and prevents over-stimulation of the points, which could lead to excess toxins being released, causing the mother to feel ill. It is wise to avoid areas where the skin is irritated, burnt or recently scarred for obvious reasons, and acupressure points situated over lymph glands should be touched only very lightly to avoid pain and discomfort.

Reflexology   Reflexology is a manual treatment in which the feet represent a map of the body so that by working on specific parts of the feet other areas of the body can be treated. Although it is not known how reflexology works, the Eastern theory is that it involves similar principles to acupressure: by working on the meridians in the feet, treatment is directed to related zones in the body. The Western theory relates it to the nervous system, with nerve endings in the feet being manipulated which then influence other parts of the body. Although reflexology is not a standard element of aromatherapy massage, and does not normally involve the use of oils, it can occasionally serve as an alternative or a complement to other manual techniques used in massage (see also Tiran and Mack, 1995, Ch. 4).

Baby massage   Massage of the neonate, either by mothers or midwives, has become extremely popular recently as it is recognized that touch can be so soothing. There are many reports of midwives and health visitors establishing classes at which parents can learn and become confident in massaging their infants (Adamson, 1993; Bowers-Clarke, 1993; Isherwood, 1994), although it must be stressed that professionals should be adequately trained to offer this service.

The benefits of regular baby massage, especially in preterm infants, have been shown to be an enhanced parent–infant relationship (White-Traut and Nelson, 1988), maintenance of body temperature (Johanson et al., 1992), enhanced maturation and growth (Kuhn et al., 1991; Field et al., 1986) and improved prognosis for intellectual development (Adamson-Macedo, 1993).

For the parents, physical contact with the baby will incresae their confidence in general handling and can indirectly help to relax them—fretful babies lead to distressed mothers and this is in turn transmitted back to the baby so that the whole episode becomes a vicious circle. Teaching parents to massage their baby is one of the easiest and most pleasant means of achieving a good family relationship and should be promoted from birth. Parents can be encouraged to follow the bath time with a few valuable minutes spent stroking the baby, perhaps as they apply baby lotion, talcum powder or oil.

After feeding, the mother could maintain contact with her baby, just gently stroking the back and head, rather than concentrating on the outmoded 'winding', which is still suggested on occasions. If any investigations such as phenylketonuria or serum bilirubin tests are required, the mother could sit with the infant on her knee and massage accessible areas of the body, or simply hold the baby's hand. Baby massage classes provide an opportunity for parents not only to develop further their relationship with their child but offer valuable access to a midwife or health visitor, who may achieve more in less time than seeing mothers individually at routine child health clinics.

Even when a neonate is seriously ill, the parents could insert a hand into the incubator and maintain contact by stroking the baby's head, hand or leg. This does not have to be intrusive and interfere with any necessary technology, but can facilitate for the parents a sense of belonging and of being involved in the care of their baby. Initially it will require the midwives to suggest various ways of touching the baby, but will probably occur spontaneously if parents observe the staff also enjoying regular contact with the child. This will serve as a form of 'permission giving' to parents who may feel afraid to touch the baby—a baby who seems to belong more to the staff than to themselves. Midwives and neonatal nurses should constantly be considering ways in which they can demonstrate the benefits of touch, and set an example to the parents.

Views on whether preterm infants should be touched or left undisturbed have changed radically in the past few years, but there may be occasions when massage is contraindicated. These include hyperpyrexial infants, in whom the vasodilatory effects of massage could severely compromise the condition; babies whose cerebral condition is so unstable that tactile communication may initiate a fit; those with major cardiac conditions; and infected neonates. Common sense on the part of the staff will help them to decide whether an individual baby seems well enough to receive some form of massage or touch therapy.

Application through the skin: in water

Essential oils can be administered in the bath water, providing a pleasant-smelling and relaxing experience. The oils should be diluted to the required dosage (see The Art of Blending below) and should not be dropped into the water neat. This is because oil will float on the surface of the water and, if the neat oil then comes in contact with the skin, it may cause irritation. Therefore, the oils can be blended with either the normal base oil or in another fluid which facilitates dispersion, such as full cream milk, very mild shampoo or even vodka (although this seems rather a waste of vodka!).

If an aromatic bath is considered appropriate, the essential oils should be added to the water after the bath is filled, and dispersed thoroughly; if the oils are added while the hot tap is running, the steam will cause the volatile oils to evaporate. Alternatively sprigs of fresh herbs can be hung under the stream of water as it fills the bath.

The temperature and depth of the water will depend on the purpose for which the bath is being taken. If the object is to aid relaxation and induce sleep, a deep but tepid bath is best; to invigorate, a short, hot, shallower bath can be effective—but very hot water can be debilitating if the bath is prolonged. Pregnant women should be discouraged from very hot baths in any case, as their temperature is already raised as a result of increased blood volume.

For a general de-stressing soak it is pleasant to be able to submerge under deep water, although this may not always be practical. Mothers wishing to labour in the bath may have essential oils added if the membranes are intact, but once ruptured the water should be changed, and if delivery takes place in the bath no essential oils should be used. This is to avoid the risk to the baby's eyes of coming in contact with the oils. Garland (1995, p. 122) states that in her unit no other means of analgesia is used when women labour in the bath, as the water itself is intended as a pain reliever, although Lichy and Herzberg (1993, p. 119) suggest that the addition of 'a few drops' of essential oil to the bath water can be helpful. This author advocates a cautious approach to the use of essential oils during water birth, in line with Garland's comments.

Where localized wounds such as caesarean section or episiotomy are to be bathed, the water level must obviously be high enough to cover the afflicted area, although a bidet could also be used for perineal bathing. Foot baths are a practical method of providing aromatherapy as they enable the mother to receive essential oils systemically yet use little water and do not require much super-vision. One often-quoted anecdote, which indicates how quickly essential oils are transported around the body, is that of a test in which essential oil of garlic was applied to the subject's feet, and within 20 minutes the odour was detectable on his breath (see also Part 1).

Compresses Compresses can be made by soaking a cloth (a sanitary towel is especially good) in the water to which the essential oils have previously been added; the excess is squeezed out and the compress applied to the affected area. This is a particularly effective and efficient method during labour when the mother may wish to receive aromatherapy in a form other than massage and yet feels unable to climb in and out of a bath, or if bathrooms in the maternity unit are all in use. Compresses applied to the suprapubic and sacral areas during the first stage using oils such as clary sage can be comforting and analgesic, and in the second and third stages lavender and/or jasmine may enhance uterine action.

Vulval washes Vulval washes may be used for infections, leucorrhoea and as a general hygiene measure; tea tree–soaked tampons are excellent for treating vaginal thrush. Douches are recommended by many aromatherapy authorities but should be used with caution during the childbearing period and avoided once the membranes have ruptured and in the puerperium to minimize the dangers of fluid embolism entering the circulation via the placental site.

Although it is acceptable for essential oils to be used in jacuzzis and saunas, these methods of administration are contraindicated in pregnancy. Jacuzzis should be avoided because of the risk of embolism if water enters the vagina; saunas will raise the mother's temperature to a level that could adversely affect the fetus.

Application via the respiratory tract Inhalation of essential oils is a logical means of administration for conditions specifically affecting the respiratory tract, although, as with other local applications, the effects will eventually be systemic. Where mothers are suffering from a cold, influenza, sinus congestion or postoperative chest infection, essential oils can be added to hot water and given via a traditional inhalation apparatus or simply by leaning over the bowl with a towel covering the head to direct the vapours towards the nostrils. This latter method can also be used as a facial sauna in cases of acne or other skin conditions.

Various items of equipment are now available to facilitate diffusion of essential oils (Fig. 6.2). Some are decorative pots incorporating a heat source such as a night-light candle which helps the volatile essential oils to evaporate. However, those with a naked flame contravene institutional health and safety regulations and should never be used in the maternity unit. If a mother chooses to use one in the home she should be advised about safe positioning,

Fig 6.2 Equipment for vaporizing essential oils.

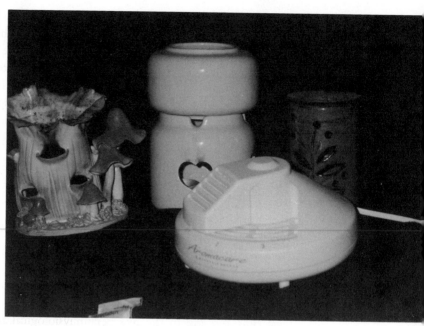

remembering that in labour she may inadvertently move an arm or leg and knock it over if it is too close.

Other devices for vaporizing essential oils include small porcelain rings. Two or three essential oil drops (without water) are added to the ring, which is rested on an upturned light bulb for its heat source. Some authorities suggest adding essential oils to a humidifier (McGilvery and Reed, 1993, p. 13), or resting a bowl of water containing the essential oils on top of the radiator.

Electrical vaporizers are the most suitable for use in the maternity unit, and despite the additional cost are safer and more durable. They are useful in the labour ward where mothers are normally in single rooms, but should be turned on intermittently; this is to prevent the aroma from becoming overpowering and to avoid 'aroma immunity'. Ten minutes of vaporization in each hour will probably be sufficient; on no account should the vaporizer be left on constantly.

Room sprays can be made using ten drops of a blend of essential oils in approximately 200 ml of water. Lemon essential oil makes a refreshing room deodorizer and freshener. Pot pourri can also, of course, be used, with the essential oils being added every few days.

For mothers who have difficulty in sleeping, two drops of an essential oil such as lavender or camomile, according to preference, can be put directly on to the pillow; likewise, fretful babies can benefit from the application of *one* drop of camomile oil on the sheet near their heads. For pregnant women with sinus congestion, two drops of tea tree or marjoram oil on a cotton handkerchief and sniffed at intervals can provide relief.

The art of blending essential oils

The choice of essential oils to be used for a mother depends on several factors. The therapeutic requirements are obviously of prime importance, together with an acknowledgement of any contraindications to specific oils. For example, two oils which together are effective in treating headache are lavender and peppermint, but while lavender may be used towards term in small doses, the safety of peppermint at any time during pregnancy is debatable, so it would be wiser to use lavender alone.

Essential oil chemicals have both physiological and psychological effects, the latter as a result of the aromas working directly on the brain through the olfactory organ (see Chapter 4). To continue the example of the woman with a headache, in the first or second trimester even lavender oil would be contraindicated as there is currently no evidence to demonstrate whether or not its purported emmenagogic action can induce miscarriage. A gentle oil such as mandarin or orange is not identified specifically as an analgesic, but its relaxing and uplifting qualities, especially when administered via massage, may be a suitable alternative for a tension headache.

It is perfectly acceptable to select a single essential oil in a carrier, but up to five oils may be blended together if this is justified. Within midwifery the use of only one oil would assist in identifying any untoward side-effects, enabling those that adversely affect a mother to be avoided. Essential oils are known to work synergistically, however; in other words, the total effect of a blend is more than the sum of its parts, with one oil enhancing the action of another.

Dosage   The dosage of essential oils for use in pregnancy and labour should be no more than 1–2 per cent for massage, preferably less in pregnancy; and 4 per cent for baths. For newly delivered mothers a 2–3 per cent blend can be used (4–6 per cent in baths), and neonates should never receive more than a 1 per cent blend at any time. All essential oils should be added to a base or carrier oil, and the amount calculated as follows.

For each 5 millilitres (ml) of base oil the number of drops added will be the same as the percentage blend required, e.g. for a 2 per cent blend, two drops are added to 5 ml base oil; for a 3 per cent blend three drops are needed, and so on. When a 1.5 per cent blend is favoured, the amount of base oil needs to be doubled, as it is not possible to add half drops of essential oil, i.e. three drops of essential oil are added to 10 ml base oil to make a 1.5 per cent blend.

The total number of drops must never exceed that required when only one oil is used, so that if a 2 per cent mix using lavender and mandarin is wanted, only one drop of each is added to 5 ml base oil. This does, however, pose a challenge to the aromatherapist, for how does she decide on the most appropriate balance of essential oils when more than one is used?

Let us consider a mother with postnatal urinary tract infection, for which the midwife-aromatherapist decides to use a 2.5 per cent blend of bergamot and sandalwood, both of which have an affinity for the urinary tract. This would mean that to 10 ml of base oil five drops of essential oil should be added—but in what proportion? It is probable that the practitioner would choose two drops of one oil and three drops of the other; from an aromatic viewpoint it would be preferable for sandalwood to be in the greater proportion for this oil takes a while to warm up and become a noticeable aroma.

In cases where several essential oils are used together, it is partly a knowledge of each oil's therapeutic properties, partly client preference and partly experience of the art of blending which dictates the selection of the proportions of the oils. Essential oil molecules begin the process of evaporation as soon as they are exposed to the air and continue for varying lengths of time, according to the volatility of the oil and other factors that may accelerate the process. This degeneration causes a constantly changing chemical composition as some constituents evaporate faster than others (see Part 1).

Consequently the aromas alter, albeit subtly. Certainly the initial fresh aroma will eventually give way to one which is the main 'theme' of the essential oil blend. This will be followed at a later stage by a different, more persistent, odour which will endure for anything up to 8 hours.

The 'notes' system of blending   These chemical changes led to the development by a perfumer, Septimus Piesse, in the nineteenth century of a system of 'notes' to facilitate the creation of harmonious perfumes. There are now more sophisticated methods in use but the principles still apply and can be adapted for creativity in aromatherapy.

As a general rule, essential oils extracted from the tops of plants—the flowers and fruit—are the 'top' notes, providing fresh fruity aromas immediately noticeable on blending but relatively short-lived. These include the citrus essences and others with distinctive sharp aromas such as lemongrass, ginger and eucalyptus.

Essential oils from the whole plant, leaves and stems, i.e. the middle part of the plant, constitute the 'middle' notes, which are often used as the main therapeutic oil of the blend. This includes most of the herbal oils. The 'base' notes are those oils extracted from the base of the plant, e.g. the roots, seeds, bark and wood. They have aromas which emerge only after warming of the oil but which linger the longest; they include carrot seed, sandalwood and rosewood.

A useful comparison to help midwives understand this concept of notes is to consider the drug Syntometrine, given intramuscularly to aid placental separation. Within this drug the oxytocin component works rapidly to initiate an almost immmediate uterine contraction and to force the placenta to separate from the decidua, but its action is short-lived. The work of this 'synergistic' blend of drugs is then taken over by ergometrine which takes several minutes to have an effect but whose action is then sustained to prevent uterine relaxation and consequent haemorrhage.

Other methods of blending Many aromatherapists use the notes system of blending to help their choice of essential oils. Another method is to blend oils that originate from the same family, for example citrus essences (Rutaceae family) or herbal oils (Labiatae family). Oils that contain the same chemical constituents marry well, such as those containing the aldehyde citronellal (eucalyptus, melissa, mandarin and lemongrass), while on the other hand some chemical constituents 'compete' aromatically, making the resultant blend unacceptable.

Essential oils from the same parts of plants enhance each other, for example those from fruits or from woods. A few essential oils, such as lavender and rose, are extremely versatile and blend well with a large number of other oils, whereas others have such a distinctive aroma that their flexibility is limited, e.g. garlic.

Much of the art of blending essential oils comes from an instinctive feel for what is right—and some therapists are better at blending than others. One of the easiest ways of selecting oils is to remove the bottle tops from those being considered and waft them slowly past

Constituent	Odour	Essential oil
Aldehydes		
Cinnamic aldehyde	Cinnamon-like	Cinnamon
Citral	Citrus, lemon	Mandarin
Citronellal	Citrus, rose-like	Lemon
Esters		
Benzyl acetate	Floral, fruity	Ylang ylang
Bornyl acetate	Camphorous	Rosemary
Geranyl acetate	Sweet, rose-like, fruity	Lemongrass
Linalyl acetate	Light, herbal, slightly fruity	Clary sage
Neryl acetate	Sweet, rose-like, fruity	Neroli
Alcohols		
Borneol	Woody, camphorous	Rosemary
Cedrol	Faintly woody	Cypress
Citronellol	Rich, floral, rose-like	Geranium
Linalol	Floral, woody, slightly spicy	Basil
Menthol	Fresh, minty	Peppermint
Nerol	Sweet, floral, slightly seaweedy	Neroli
Ketones		
Camphor	Fresh, warm, minty	Marjoram
Fenchone	Warm, camphorous	Fennel
Menthone	Minty, slightly woody	Peppermint
Thujone	Strong, herbal, camphorous	Sage
Phenols		
Carvacrol	Tar-like, herbal, spicy	Thyme
Estragol	Sweet, herbal, aniseed-like	Fennel
Eugenol	Spicy, clove-like	Marjoram
Methyl chavicol	Similar to estragol	Basil
Safrole	Warm, spicy, woody	Nutmeg
Oxides		
1.8 Cineole	Eucalyptus-like	Eucalyptus
Monoterpenes		
Camphene	Camphorous	Juniper
Limonene	Weak citrus	Grapefruit
Myrcene	Sweet, balsamic	Black pepper
Phellandrene	Citrus, spicy, woody	Frankincense
Pinene	Woody, pine-like	Petitgrain
Sesquiterpenes		
α-Terpinene	Fresh, citrus-like	Tea tree
β-Bisabolene	Balsamic, spicy	Camomile
Sabinene	Spicy, woody, herbal	Juniper

the nostrils of both the client and the practitioner. This will give an idea of whether the oils enhance or compete with each other, but it is really only with continued practice that individuals become 'nasally tuned in' and adept at selecting oils that blend well.

Many of the main chemical constituents of essential oils have now been identified, through scientific analysis, as having specific odour classifications. There are also many less commonly found or as yet undiscovered chemicals still to be classified, and a few examples are given in Table 6.4.

Chapter 7

Using Essential Oils in Midwifery Practice

It has been emphasized elsewhere in this book that the benefits of using essential oils for the childbearing woman and her infant must be balanced by a thorough working knowledge of the potential hazards of the substances (see Part 1). Aromatherapy is as safe a system of care as any other when used by appropriately trained and experienced practitioners, but in a similar way to pharmacological preparations is open either to inadvertent or intentional misuse.

However, there are many situations within midwifery practice when aromatherapy can be of great value, and this section addresses those occasions. In some instances it may be appropriate to use essential oils in conjunction with conventional care, perhaps to relieve stress; in others, aromatherapy is used as an alternative, either as essential oils or as a herbal infusion. In some cases, manual techniques including shiatsu and reflexology may be appropriate, with or without essential oils, and suggestions are made for incorporating these into the care of the mothers and babies; where other complementary therapies may be more effective, these have not been dealt with here and midwives and aromatherapists are referred to the list of further reading for additional information.

Appetite changes   Expectant and newly delivered mothers may find that their appetite changes. This may be a reduced desire to eat, perhaps due to physiological effects such as nausea, or an increase in appetite (probably because oestrogen is an appetite stimulant), and occasionally cravings or pica, thought to be due to certain dietary deficiencies.

Essential oil of bergamot may act as an appetite regulator (Davis, 1988, p. 34), making it useful for either a loss of or an increase in appetite. As far as is known, this oil is safe to use during pregnancy and could be given to the mother to add to her bath. Small amounts of bergamot are found in Earl Grey tea, although some women dislike the taste of tea in pregnancy.

Essential oils of marjoram, thyme and melissa are suggested as appetite stimulants by Ryman (1991, p. 233), while Valnet (1982, p. 200) also recommends caraway, camomile, coriander, hyssop, juniper, nutmeg, origanum, sage and tarragon; although these are not suitable for use in pregnancy some such as camomile may be helpful postpartum. Sage, however, is definitely contraindicated during the childbearing phase, even after delivery while lochia are being discharged, because of its tendency to induce or increase uterine bleeding, and should probably be avoided altogether in women of reproductive years unless under the control of an experienced aromatherapist.

Fresh lemon or lime juice can assist in removing a sour taste from the mouth, especially if the expectant mother has been vomiting; inhaling essential oil of lime may reduce pica or relieve excess salivation, which can sometimes be a distressing problem. Ginger and lemongrass are also thought to stimulate the appetite. Fennel, often quoted as an appetite stimulant, is not suitable for administration in pregnancy.

Backache   Backache in pregnancy is extremely common owing to the influence of the relaxin and progesterone hormones and the consequent lumbar lordosis that occurs as compensation for the increasing abdominal growth and weight.

Simple massage with base oil may be sufficient but can be enhanced by the use of some essential oils, although those most appropriate for dealing with muscular pains are contraindicated in early pregnancy: lavender, marjoram and rosemary. These can be used in labour, however, and may facilitate uterine action when an occipito-posterior position of the fetus is the cause of lumbosacral pain. (Rosemary should not be used if the mother is hypertensive.) Clary sage may also be helpful where there is an occipito-posterior position, as it will act as an overall analgesic and assist in relaxing the mother.

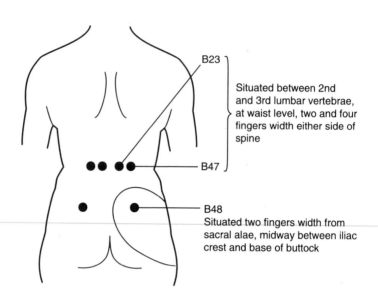

Fig 7.1 Shiatsu
points to relieve
backache.

Black pepper in small doses, perhaps combined with a relaxing oil such as mandarin, neroli or petitgrain, will be warming and can relieve acute pain. Alternatively a warm bath to which has been added a few drops of a de-stressing oil may be sufficient.

Pressure applied to the shiatsu points may be effective in relieving symptoms; sciatica and lumbosacral pain can be eased by pressure to the B23, B47 and B48 points (Fig. 7.1), although these points might be quite tender to touch at first.

Reflexology to the foot zones for the spine can also help and a full reflexology treatment may relax the mother sufficiently to work indirectly on the pain. It must be stressed, however, that these suggestions will not treat the cause, and any mother who suffers perpetual backache during pregnancy or postnatally should be referred to an osteopath.

Geraldine's labour was long and painful due to an occipito-posterior position of the fetus which caused her considerable backache. The midwife suggested a variety of postural changes in the early phase and encouraged Geraldine to relax in a bath to which had been added essential oils of lavender and clary sage. As labour progressed Geraldine wished to remain on the bed, although she was unable to make herself comfortable. Compresses of clary sage, lavender and mandarin were applied to the suprapubic and sacral areas, and helped a little. The midwife also massaged Geraldine's sacrum and applied acupressure to the relevant shiatsu points. Although these ministrations did not relieve the backache completely, Geraldine did at least feel more relaxed and nurtured, and at times was able to doze between contractions.

Blood pressure   Several essential oils can have an effect on the blood pressure, either by raising or lowering it (Table 7.1). The choice of oils will of course depend upon the desired effect; it is vital that midwives are aware of these effects, and that aromatherapists have a thorough understanding of changes in the blood pressure during pregnancy, labour and the puerperium, and the potential dangers of the oils they may choose.

If a pregnant woman's blood pressure is raised, any aromatherapy treatment offered by the midwife must be with the knowledge and approval of the obstetrician because of the risk of interaction with hypotensive drugs and the dangers of eclampsia. It may be, however, that the consultant is willing to try aromatherapy treatment for the mother, and there are reported cases of successful treatment of gestational hypertension using oils such as rosewood (McArdle, 1992). Rosewood was also used by Waymouth (1992) for essential hypertension.

Essential oils that have been found to lower blood pressure include many that are not to be used during pregnancy such as celery, clary sage, lavender (although lavender could be used towards term, and both lavender and clary sage may be used in labour), marjoram and melissa. Lemon, mandarin, neroli and ylang ylang can be used safely and, combined with massage, may have the desired effect. Garlic is also a hypotensor and the mother could be advised to eat plenty of whole cloves of garlic in her diet. (Using them whole in cooking increases the amount of therapeutic ingredient but does not seem to overpower the flavour or leave an after-taste or breath odour.)

If the hypertension is thought to be exacerbated by stress and tension, any of the safe anti-anxiety oils could be used with massage

Table 7.1
Essential oils that affect blood pressure

Hypotensives				
Celery	Clary sage	Garlic	Lavender	Lemon
Marjoram	Melissa	Rosewood	Ylang ylang	

Hypertensives			
Hyssop	Rosemary	Sage	Thyme

to help relax the mother, while simple massage with a base oil could be carried out by the partner. Other manual techniques could be employed to ease associated symptoms such as nausea and vomiting, headaches and ankle oedema, while abdominal massage may calm the fetus.

It is obvious that, while the above-mentioned essential oils can be used therapeutically in cases where the blood pressure needs to be reduced, these same oils would be contraindicated in women with existing low blood pressure. This would apply to all the oils, with the exception of mandarin, lemon and garlic, during the second trimester of pregnancy when there is a physiological lowering of the blood pressure, and also during labour if the mother is receiving epidural anaesthesia which can lead to hypotension.

Conversely there are essential oils that raise the blood pressure and could theoretically be of use in women whose blood pressure is excessively low. These oils are normally contraindicated during pregnancy as they are emmenagogic—hyssop, sage, thyme and rosemary—but it may be appropriate to use rosemary with caution near term and in labour.

If a mother suffers from postural hypotension it may be possible to teach her a shiatsu first-aid technique, applying pressure to the K1 point on the centre of the foot where the ball of the foot joins the arch (Fig. 7.2).

Fig 7.2 K1 shiatsu first-aid point for postural hypotension.

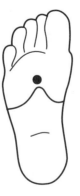

K1 point – situated on soles of feet, at base of the ball, midway between the two pads of the feet

On the third day after delivery Sandra was very tearful, mainly due to the fact that her ankles and feet had swollen to such an extent that the skin was excessively tight; she was constipated, and felt tired and depressed. Her blood pressure had been raised antenatally and returned to normal after the birth, but her distress seemed to be the cause of it increasing again.

On entering the room the aromatherapist was confronted by Sandra in floods of tears, but after administering Bach Rescue Remedy and gently talking to Sandra she calmed down sufficiently to agree to a foot massage.

The aromatherapist used a combination of ylang ylang (to relax the mother and decrease the blood pressure), jasmine (good for postnatal depression and 'blues'), mandarin (refreshing and calming) and cypress (to reduce the oedema), and commenced firm bimanual upwards massage of the feet, ankles and lower legs. Within 5 minutes one foot was signifi-cantly improved, the skin felt looser and more comfortable, and Sandra was beginning to relax. Once the oedema had been dealt with, the therapist was able to incorporate reflexology to the arches of the feet, the zones for the gastrointestinal tract, to treat the constipation, and then repeat the treatment on the other foot. By the end of the 20-minute session, Sandra's feet looked almost normal, she felt soporific and calm, and her diastolic blood pressure had reduced to normal limits. The next day she reported a successful bowel action, she felt much more relaxed and was normotensive once again.

Breast care Breast and nipple self-massage may be suggested antenatally to mothers, both to prepare them for labour and breastfeeding, and to stimulate lactation after delivery. Breast massage is performed gently, working towards the nipple; it encourages the mother to become accustomed to handling her breasts before lactation. Massage from the axilla to the nipple can facilitate milk flow and prevent stasis.

Nipple massage, rolling the nipple between thumb and forefinger, can be carried out daily in the last 4 weeks of pregnancy to stimulate oxytocin production which will help to ripen the cervix in prepara-tion for labour, harden the nipples for breastfeeding and promote a good supply of milk. Mothers should be advised to massage only one nipple at a time, for about 5 minutes, as bilateral stimulation could precipitate hypertonic uterine action.

Aromatherapy oils or herbal teas can help the mother who is breastfeeding. Essential oils classified as galactogues (increasing lacta-tion) can be used to stimulate milk production and include aniseed, basil, caraway, dill, fennel, lemongrass and jasmine. Any direct application of essential oils to the breasts in massage or in the bath

Fig 7.3 (a) Foot reflex
zone therapy to
stimulate lactation.

(a)

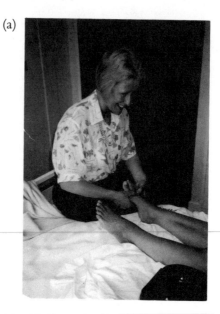

Fig 7.3 (b) Hand
reflex zones to massage
to encourage lactation.
(From Tiran &
Mack, 1995).

(b)

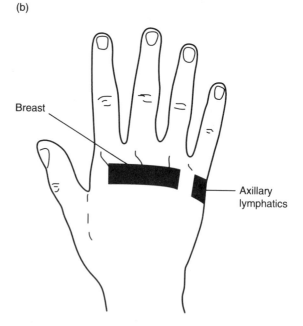

Fig 7.3 (c) Shiatsu points to stimulate lactation.

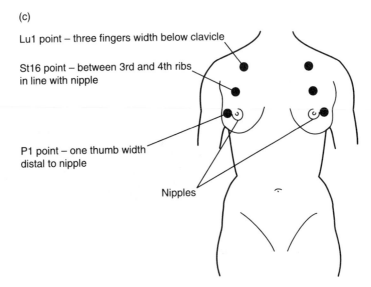

(c)

Lu1 point – three fingers width below clavicle

St16 point – between 3rd and 4th ribs in line with nipple

P1 point – one thumb width distal to nipple

Nipples

should be rinsed off before putting the baby to the breast to avoid ingestion, but many of these, notably fennel, dill or jasmine, can be drunk as a tea throughout the puerperium.

When the milk supply is poor, stimulation of the reflexology breast zones on the feet can be attempted (Fig. 7.3(a)). Rather than carry out specific reflexology techniques, the midwife can gently massage these areas and advise the mother to rub the corresponding hand zones intermittently (Fig. 7.3(b)). There is a theory that women who have had an intravenous infusion, sited in the dorsum of the hand during labour, may have impaired lactation, and this would be well worth investigating. The shiatsu points P1 and St16 can also be stimulated to promote lactation (Fig. 7.3(c)).

For engorgement of the breasts, the application of cabbage leaves produces, in many women, spectacular results. Dark green cabbage leaves are wiped clean and cooled in the refrigerator then applied to engorged breasts. Often within seconds the leaves become wet, when they should be removed and replaced with new leaves, this process being repeated until relief is obtained. Women who have employed this method of relieving engorgement are amazed at the results despite their initial scepticism, and it provides an inexpensive means of treatment without any known side-effects.

Suppression of lactation has been achieved with jasmine flowers. Shrivastav *et al.* (1988) demonstrated a reduction in serum prolactin levels in women who had had jasmine flowers applied to the breasts, and the earlier work of Abraham *et al.* (1979) suggested that pituitary inhibition occurs as a result of an olfactory pathway to the hypothalamus. This does bring into question the use of jasmine to stimulate lactation, although it may be that the essential oil acts as a *regulator*, not specifically as a stimulant or suppressant.

Similarly, Tisserand (1992, p. 298) suggested that geranium may be useful as a means of reducing the flow of milk, yet Worwood (1991, p. 282) has advocated geranium to stimulate lactation. Alternative suppressants include peppermint: Davis (1988, p. 62) recommends a cold compress soaked in water and oil of peppermint, but again advises washing the breasts before feeding the baby.

Sore nipples may respond to the direct application of geranium leaves or the use of a cream to which has been added a few drops of geranium essential oil. Calendula essential oil is recommended by some authorities but there are several proprietary brands of calendula creams which can be used rather than making one's own. Camomile has also been used both in essential oil form and as a proprietary cream (Kamillosan). A simple home remedy for sore nipples is to steep camomile teabags in boiled water, drain, cool and then apply them to the nipples, keeping them in place with the bra.

If the mother shows signs and symptoms of mastitis or a developing breast abscess, a compress of tea tree oil is the most effective method of combating infection; alternatively geranium essential oil can be used.

Bruising

By far the best treatment for severe bruising, particularly of the perineum and/or buttocks following delivery, is arnica, a homoeopathic preparation and one of the few that is universally appropriate for trauma. It is available in both cream and tablet form, although the cream should not be applied to an open wound such as a perineal suture line. Tablets should be taken immediately after the birth and at 4-hourly intervals thereafter until the symptoms subside, usually about 3 days. Arnica is included here because it should be the first line of treatment and a normal part of midwifery care. Midwives should take action to introduce it into their units by stimulating discussion with medical and managerial colleagues and presenting sufficient evidence to convince them of the benefits of a trial period. Homoeopathic arnica can be given safely in pregnancy, for example when a large contusion has developed after a difficult venepuncture, but the essential oil is contraindicated completely in aromatherapy.

There are some essential oils that can be valuable for bruising, the safest of which is lavender, from the third trimester onwards. If this is used in a bath or bidet it may also help perineal healing following delivery, while oil of black pepper added to the bidet or massaged into the skin can relieve the discomfort of bruised buttocks. Other oils effective in dealing with bruising are not considered safe during pregnancy and include fennel, hyssop and sage (Valnet, 1982, p. 202) and marjoram, mint and parsley (Ryman, 1991, p. 242), although marjoram could be applied postnatally.

Conjunctivitis

Most commonly, midwives will observe conjunctivitis in the neonate. As the eye is a sensitive area of the body, it is necessary to ensure that medical advice is sought as soon as possible to eliminate more serious problems, but where the baby (or mother) suffers from true conjunctivitis aromatherapy principles can be of use. It is important to remember, however, that essential oils should *never* be used on the eyes even when they are well diluted. The simplest and safest management is to irrigate the eye with a solution of camomile tea, with its soothing, anti-inflammatory and antiseptic properties. Rose is thought to be effective and can be applied in the form of an eye compress soaked in rosewater, but camomile is usually more easily available.

Constipation and colic

A variety of factors contribute to the high incidence of constipation in pregnant and newly delivered mothers, and in their infants. The action of progesterone in relaxing the gastrointestinal tract and slowing peristalsis provides a physiological reason for gestational difficulties with defaecation, often compounded by the unnecessary use of regular iron adminstration, although this practice, fortunately, is on the decline. A high intake of tea (tannin) will also exacerbate the condition. The traditional practice of restricting food intake during labour (although less so now), together with poor postnatal nutrition for many mothers in hospital, adds to the problem, as does the reflex inhibition from which many mothers suffer if there is perineal trauma.

The easiest and most effective treatment is firm clockwise abdominal massage, carried out for about 5 minutes, and/or clockwise massage of the arches of the feet. This latter works on the reflex zones to the gastrointestinal tract and may be easier on heavily pregnant women. It is not feasible to perform abdominal massage

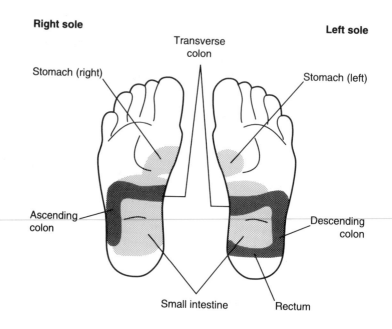

Fig 7.4 Reflex zones for the gastrointestinal tract. Note the direction of the intestines: clockwise massage of the foot arches will treat constipation.

on a mother who has had a Caesarean section, but *gentle* clockwise massage of the foot arches may produce results (Fig. 7.4).

The mother can be directed to perform intermittent self-shiatsu on the CV6 point. She should lie on her back and press deeply to a depth of about one inch, then maintain the pressure for a few minutes whilst breathing deeply. The LI11 point can also be worked, and postnatally the LI4 point, although this is contraindicated during pregnancy (Fig. 7.5).

If the neonate becomes constipated the same gentle clockwise abdominal and foot arch massage can be carried out, by either the midwife or the mother. Similarly when the baby suffers from colic, abdominal massage will stimulate peristalsis so that the air bubbles will be pushed along the intestines and expelled via the rectum. It is best to show the mother how to do it herself, for a fretful baby often leads to a distressed mother, and the action of performing the massage may help in calming her. Camomile tea can be given on a teaspoon, flavoured with honey if necessary.

If essential oils are used to treat constipation, mandarin, tangerine, orange, lemon, lemongrass, lime, grapefruit, or perhaps benzoin, in any combination, can help (Table 7.2). Tisserand (1992, p. 300) includes bergamot and black pepper, which may be used in pregnancy, and camphor, cardamon, clary sage, fennel, hyssop, juniper,

Fig 7.5 Shiatsu
points for constipation.

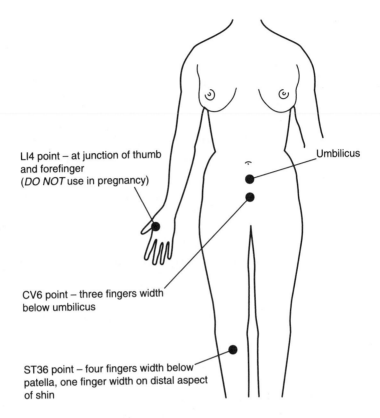

LI4 point – at junction of thumb
and forefinger
(*DO NOT* use in pregnancy)

Umbilicus

CV6 point – three fingers width
below umbilicus

ST36 point – four fingers width below
patella, one finger width on distal aspect
of shin

lavender, marjoram, myrrh, peppermint and rosemary, which may
not. (Lavender, juniper, marjoram and rosemary may be used in
small doses near term, but as there are safer oils for the treatment
of constipation it would be advisable to refrain from using these until
the puerperium.)

Expectant and newly delivered mothers may like to drink camomile tea and to increase the amount of citrus fruit in the diet.
Postnatally a massage with a blend of orange, grapefruit, nutmeg
and camomile, applied to the abdomen in a clockwise direction and
to the sacral area of the lower back, can work wonders.

Table 7.2 Essential oils for constipation and colic				
Benzoin	Black pepper	Grapefruit	Lemongrass	Lime
Mandarin	Marjoram	Rosemary	Sweet orange	Tangerine

Depression Hormonal upheavals, especially in the postnatal period, can lead to depression of varying severity. Many women experience the 'blues' about 3–4 days after delivery and quickly recover. Others develop the condition within the first 6 weeks after the birth; some will have a low-grade depression which they are able to deal with themselves, and some will require short- or long-term psychiatric support. A few women develop depression during pregnancy, although many more feel a variety of emotions such as anxiety, fear and stress.

The emotional symptoms of depression may take many forms, including fear and anxiety, panic, paranoia, impatience, apathy and irritability, and various essential oils can be utilized to combat these symptoms (Table 7.3). Jasmine, patchouli, rose and frankincense are among the most effective, although jasmine and rose are emmenagogic, so are contraindicated during pregnancy.

Each of these oils has a rich, luxurious aroma which seems to pamper and nurture the woman, but it may be necessary to subdue the aroma by blending it with other oils, such as bergamot, camomile, sandalwood or ylang ylang. Neroli and orange blended together can be very pleasant and safe to use during pregnancy as well as after delivery, and other citrus oils can be helpful, such as grapefruit, mandarin and lime.

Tisserand (1992, p. 101) classifies oils suitable for dealing with the individual symptoms of depression, and includes basil, benzoin, bergamot, cypress, sandalwood and ylang ylang for anxiety, plus camomile, frankincense, geranium, neroli and rose for depression. Other oils suggested include juniper for associated apathy, clary sage for fear, melissa for hypersensitivity or hypochondria, lavender for irritability, panic or hysteria. Valnet (1982, p. 207) highlights camomile or neroli for nervous depressive states, while Ryman (1991, p. 265) recommends energizing herbs such as marjoram and thyme either used as the whole herb in cooking or teas, or as the essential oil rubbed into the solar plexus area below the ribs.

A full-body or back massage as a stress reliever may assist in reducing some of the negative feelings which the mother may have, or a relaxing bath containing essential oils may be preferred (see also Stress and anxiety).

Shiatsu massage of the head including the GV19, GV20, GV21, GV24.5, GB20 and B10 points can be very relaxing and relieve associated headaches, and a general reflexology treatment may also help (Fig. 7.6).

Jane was a professional woman who had recently left a demanding career. She had initially been upset when she discovered she was pregnant but

Table 7.3
Essential oils to treat
depression

Benzoin	Bergamot	Camomile	Clary sage	Frankincense	
Geranium	Juniper	Lavender	Mandarin	Marjoram	Melissa
Neroli	Patchouli	Rose	Sandalwood	Thyme	Ylang ylang

Fig 7.6 Shiatsu
points to relieve
headaches.

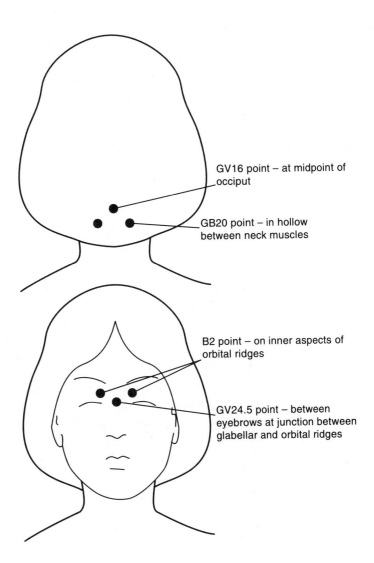

GV16 point – at midpoint of occiput

GB20 point – in hollow between neck muscles

B2 point – on inner aspects of orbital ridges

GV24.5 point – between eyebrows at junction between glabellar and orbital ridges

gradually accepted the fact, and was pleased on account of her husband who was Italian and 'over the moon' about the impending birth. However, as term approached Jane became increasingly anxious and noticeably depressed about her imagined inability to give birth and to care for the baby, and this was made worse by her husband's lack of understanding and insistence that her negative attitude was spoiling a wonderful experience for him. Eventually Jane was admitted to the antenatal ward for psychiatric referral.

The midwife-aromatherapist was able to see Jane for several consecutive days and offered a foot massage for stress relief, which she gratefully accepted. A combination of ylang ylang, mandarin and frankincense was used and Jane reported feeling much better after each massage, and was able to sleep. While this treatment was only palliative and in no way treated the cause, it did help Jane to feel calmer and gave her the opportunity to talk about her concerns.

Diarrhoea

Causative factors in cases of diarrhoea are complex, ranging from diet to stress, infective organisms and, in pregnancy, hormonal effects. Midwives will in the course of their work be able to give relevant dietary advice to mothers. Diarrhoea of infective aetiology requires medical care, although there are many essential oils that have proven antibacterial, antiviral and antifungal properties, notably tea tree. In addition to any prescribed medication, the mother could be encouraged to soak in a bath containing tea tree oil, with sufficient water to cover the abdomen, or a compress could be applied to the lower abdomen and sacrum.

When the diarrhoea is stress related, anti-anxiety essential oils should be used in synergy with antispasmodic oils. Neroli and petitgrain can be effective, while sandalwood has long been recognized in Ayurvedic medicine as a treatment for diarrhoea. Although both neroli and sandalwood are expensive, the synergistic effects of blending them together make them extremely beneficial for mothers with this problem. Camomile essential oil has also been found to have antispasmodic actions (Achterrath-Tuckermann et al., 1980). Later research (Taddei et al., 1988) compared the spasmolytic (antispasmodic) actions of peppermint, sage and rosemary oils in animals and found the effects to be similar with all three oils. Rosemary's actions were attributed to the level of pinene and borneol, and it was thought that it worked by antagonizing acetylcholine. Rosemary, therefore, may be used with caution in late pregnancy, except in women with raised blood pressure, but peppermint and sage are contraindicated.

Fig 7.7 Shiatsu points to relieve diarrhoea.

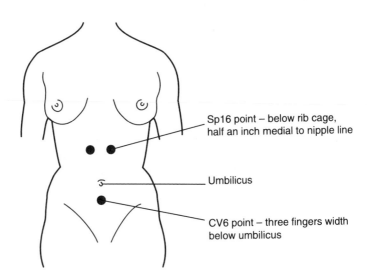

Sp16 point – below rib cage, half an inch medial to nipple line

Umbilicus

CV6 point – three fingers width below umbilicus

The essential oils can be administered as an abdominal massage, which should be *anti*clockwise to slow down peristalsis, or a compress can be applied to the suprapubic area. Similarly, anticlockwise massage of the arches of the feet will work on the reflex zones for the gastrointestinal tract, and the practitioner can incorporate shiatsu pressure to the LV2 point (Fig. 7.7). The mother can also be advised to press on the two Sp16 points on the abdomen.

If diarrhoea occurs immediately before or during labour, which is not uncommon, essential oils can be used to freshen and cleanse the mother, perhaps added to the bidet for a vulval wash; this will have the added benefit of preventing contamination by faeces of the vulval and perineal areas. Any of the above oils may be used according to the mother's preference.

Care should be taken if a baby develops diarrhoea as this may be due to gastroenteritis or an undiagnosed condition of the digestive tract. However, if it appears that the baby has simply responded adversely to something the mother may have eaten to excess (e.g. chocolate), anticlockwise abdominal massage with a 1 per cent blend of camomile or mandarin may help to slow down peristalsis. It should be stressed here that breastfed babies rarely suffer diarrhoea as a result of maternal diet and that mothers should continue to eat a well-balanced diet containing normal amounts of fruit and vegetables. Consequently practitioners should seek medical advice in cases of true neonatal diarrhoea (as opposed to loose stools).

Epilepsy   It is unlikely that midwives or aromatherapists will use essential oils to treat pregnant women with epilepsy as they will be under strict medical supervision in order to monitor the ways in which pregnancy may alter the incidence or severity of fits, and their effects on fetal and maternal wellbeing. It would indeed be irresponsible to do so without the knowledge and approval of the consultant obstetrician and physician. However, there may be some individuals in whom a fit is triggered by stress, fear, panic or anger, and it might be appropriate to offer regular massage with a safe anticonvulsive essential oil such as lavender (from the third trimester) or one that is suitable for relieving stress and anxiety, e.g. orange or ylang ylang.

Research in an epilepsy clinic with ten (non-pregnant) patients has shown that, after an initial period of regular massage with a single relaxing essential oil, patients can be taught to associate the aroma alone with a sense of relaxation and, in conjunction with auto-hypnosis, can use this as a countermeasure to prevent a fit occurring (Betts, 1994). It is interesting to note that most of these ten patients chose ylang ylang as their preferred olfactory countermeasure; in a few subjects, in whom an increase in arousal suppressed the onset of a fit, an alerting oil such as lemongrass was chosen.

It is important in maternity care to differentiate between epileptic and eclamptic fits, although the management of fits of any aetiology is the same and, during pregnancy, revolves around preserving maternal and fetal life.

When using essential oils generally for childbearing women it is necessary to be aware of oils that may initiate epileptic fits; these include rosemary, fennel, hyssop, sage and wormwood. Of these, only rosemary and fennel are likely to be used for this client group but they should be avoided in anyone with a personal or family history of epilepsy, hypertension or pre-eclampsia. Davis (1988, p. 119) suggests that minute amounts of rosemary may be helpful for epileptics, in a homoeopathic manner. This is supported by Asjes (1993), an aromatherapist experienced in the use of essential oils for epileptic children who has administered rosemary to very apathetic clients.

Epistaxis   Nosebleeds are not uncommon in pregnancy due to hypervolaemia, and capillary and vasodilatation. Essential oil of lemon acts as a haemostatic agent and can be used as a glabellary compress; alternatively a small gauze swab soaked in water to which has been added fresh lemon juice or the essential oil can be gently inserted into the nostril. If the epistaxis is associated with hypertension, lavender may also be used from the end of pregnancy.

Hair care

Pregnant and newly delivered women often experience changes in the condition or growth of their hair: some find that it becomes more greasy, others that it feels very dry; many women lose hair, especially in the months after the birth of the baby. Aromatherapy has much to offer mothers at this time, although they should be advised not to use the same essential oils consistently. The normal safeguards concerning essential oil use during pregnancy should be adhered to, for absorption through the scalp occurs as with other areas of the body.

For greasy hair the mother could use essential oil of lemon or petitgrain in early pegnancy, but, if she is not hypertensive, the most effective oil from the third trimester onwards is rosemary. Two or three drops of essential oil can be added to the rinsing water, or fresh lemon juice squeezed into the bowl; sprigs of fresh rosemary are safe to use and can be just as beneficial to the hair. A few drops of patchouli may also be used.

Camomile can be useful for hair that has been previously permed or coloured or which has become very fragile. Incidentally, most hairdressers would advise women to refrain from having a perm at this time as they are often unsuccessful, possibly due to hormonal influences.

Dry hair may respond to rosemary, geranium or sandalwood, with lavender being a useful alternative after 28 weeks' gestation. Blending the essential oils into a rich nourishing base oil such as jojoba or avocado can enhance their action.

Hair loss more commonly seems to occur in the postnatal period and can be treated with oils such as rosemary, rose, camomile, lemon, cypress, clary sage or calendula. Lime, lemon, mandarin and rosemary may help dandruff, as may thyme, although antepartum use of the latter is contraindicated.

Regular head massage, without oil, can stimulate and invigorate the scalp and may improve the condition of the hair.

Haemorrhoids

Varicose veins in the rectum and anus can be extremely painful, especially if they prolapse as they may do towards the end of pregnancy or after defaecation. Essential oils which act as an astringent and vasoconstrictor may help to relieve pain, including cypress, juniper and frankincense. These may be applied diluted as a compress, or added to a shallow bath or bidet as a local soak. Irritation and itching may be eased by using patchouli or geranium in a similar way. The mother can also be encouraged to eat plenty of garlic to aid the circulatory system in general. Ryman (1991, p. 282) recommends boiling leeks and freezing ice cubes from the cooking water, which can be rubbed on to the afflicted area for immediate relief.

Headaches

Headaches are suffered by many women in the first trimester as a result of cerebral vasodilatation, and again towards term in some, in association with hypertension. Midwives could perform a head massage (without oils) to stimulate the scalp and cerebral circulation, and to ease discomfort. The massage is performed with the midwife standing behind the mother who should be seated. A 'hairwashing' action is used to massage the scalp firmly. Massage has been compared favourably with other treatments for headaches of variable aetiology (Jenson et al., 1990).

Incorporating shiatsu can enhance the effects of simple massage, working specifically on shiatsu points GV16, GV24.5 and St3 (Fig. 7.6). In a trial by Puustjarvi et al. (1990) acupressure was used successfully in conjunction with head massage for 21 subjects with chronic tension headaches.

Other shiatsu points found on the feet can be incorporated into reflexology and include Lv3 and GB41 (Fig. 7.8). Reflexology first aid may also be effective in sedating the pain. The midwife should ascertain exactly where in the head the mother is experiencing pain and then relate this to the appropriate zone on the big toes. By gentle pressure around these zones a painful spot will be elicited; the midwife should press firmly on the epicentre of this painful spot until the pain in the toe has gone. If the headache is unilateral, only the big toe on the same side as the headache is treated; if it is bilateral then both big toes are treated (Fig. 7.8).

Miranda had suffered headaches with no identified aetiology from early in her pregnancy, and found they were relieved by resting. As she was receiving regular reflex zone therapy for stress throughout pregnancy she mentioned to her therapist that they were more frequent at about 30 weeks' gestation, although her blood pressure was normal and she had no oedema or proteinuria. The reflex zone therapist, one of the midwives in the materity unit, was able to treat Miranda for her headaches by working on her feet, with some success.

Following a normal delivery at term, Miranda again began to suffer the headaches, and this time the therapist used a combination of zone therapy and head massage. On one occasion the therapist saw Miranda while she was actually experiencing a severe headache, and applied lavender and peppermint oils to her temples, which brought a rapid response. No cause was found for the symptom and gradually the headaches subsided, probably indicating a reaction to fluctuating hormone levels, but the treatment did at least make Miranda feel more relaxed, which in itself may have helped.

Fig 7.8 Shiatsu points and reflex zones on the feet to treat headache.

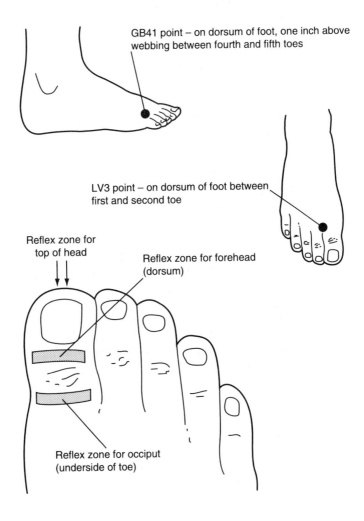

GB41 point – on dorsum of foot, one inch above webbing between fourth and fifth toes

LV3 point – on dorsum of foot between first and second toe

Reflex zone for top of head

Reflex zone for forehead (dorsum)

Reflex zone for occiput (underside of toe)

Table 7.4 Essential oils to relieve indigestion and heartburn	Black pepper Camomile (tea in pregnancy) Fennel (postnatally) Frankincense (near term) Ginger Lavender (near term) Lemon Marjoram (near term) Neroli (near term) Peppermint (postnatally) Petitgrain Sweet orange

Heartburn and indigestion

In the second and third trimesters of pregnancy, heartburn may become a problem for some women due to the increased weight and consequent pressure effects, coupled with the relaxing action of progesterone on the cardiac sphincter of the stomach. Midwives should offer the usual dietary advice but may wish to be able to help the mother by suggesting non-pharmaceutical remedies (Table 7.4).

Increased acidity in the stomach may respond to the use of lemon, either by recommending that the woman makes a lemon cordial or by gentle back and abdominal massage using the essential oil. One might assume that the acidic nature of lemon means it is contra-indicated, but it appears to work by neutralization of the citric acid, especially during digestion, resulting in the production of alkaline carbonates of calcium and potassium.

Judicious use of essential oil of black pepper in a blend with orange or mandarin can help, as may frankincense. Near term, when the use of lavender and marjoram in small amounts is not thought to be a problem, abdominal massage with a blend of these, or of lavender and camomile, can also be effective.

The carminative properties of fennel and peppermint make these two of the best plants to use for indigestion and heartburn in normal circumstances, but in pregnancy, as mentioned above, care must be taken with the essential oils until term. Teas of camomile or ginger may be best. Increasing the amount of garlic in the diet assists in reducing acidity and aiding digestion; this may depend on whether the mother likes the taste, especially at a time when the senses of taste and smell may be altered.

The use of choleretic essential oils, i.e. those that stimulate bile production, should be considered towards term or in the postnatal period. Nerol has been shown, in rats and guinea-pigs, to have choleretic effects (Rangelov et al., 1988) and is found in essential oils of neroli, petitgrain and orange.

Induction or acceleration of labour

Although not normally the province of the midwife, it may be acceptable on occasions, in consultation with the obstetricians, for manual techniques to be used in an attempt to initiate or accelerate

Fig 7.9   Shiatsu
points for labour.

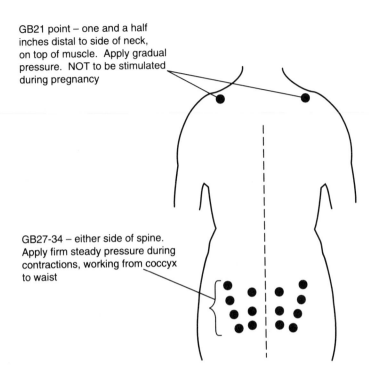

GB21 point – one and a half
inches distal to side of neck,
on top of muscle. Apply gradual
pressure. NOT to be stimulated
during pregnancy

GB27-34 – either side of spine.
Apply firm steady pressure during
contractions, working from coccyx
to waist

labour. Conversely it is important to know which techniques should
not be used during pregnancy in case they inadvertently cause
labour to commence.

Various shiatsu points can be stimulated to induce uterine action
and to relieve contraction pain, including the GB21, LI4, B67, K3
and B27–B34 points. (Fig. 7.9), although research in 1987 by Lyrenas
et al. suggests that prenatal *acupuncture*, rather than acupressure, may
prolong the duration of both pregnancy and labour. Regular
stimulation of the B67 point using the acupuncture technique of
moxibustion has also been shown to be effective in changing a
breech to a cephalic presentation (Beal, 1992; Budd, 1992).

Reflexology to the foot zones for the uterus and the pituitary
gland can be stimulated to enhance uterine action before, during or
after delivery; it can be a particularly effective treatment for retained
placenta, especially in situations such as a home birth where there
may not be access to additional drugs (Fig. 7.10).

Any of the essential oils which enhance uterine action could
theoretically be administered in an attempt to initiate contractions,
although it is likely that these will be used to accelerate labour once

Fig 7.10
Reflexology for
labour.

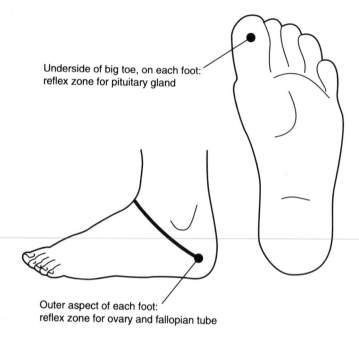

Underside of big toe, on each foot:
reflex zone for pituitary gland

Outer aspect of each foot:
reflex zone for ovary and fallopian tube

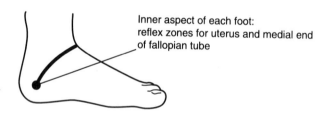

Inner aspect of each foot:
reflex zones for uterus and medial end
of fallopian tube

established. Lavender and jasmine are effective for this purpose. Raspberry leaf tea is advocated by herbalists to tone the uterus before, during and after labour. It may be drunk daily from mid-pregnancy, gradually increasing the amount, and should assist in ripening the cervix, coordinating uterine action in labour and aiding involution in the puerperium.

Insomnia and tiredness

Two of the most commonly used essential oils for helping people to sleep are camomile and lavender, but both of these are contraindicated in early pregnancy, although camomile tea may be drunk before retiring from about 24 weeks' gestation. Lavender has been shown to be effective in both inducing and prolonging sleep (Hardy, 1991; Henry *et al.*, 1994). Both of these oils can be offered to women in the postnatal period, although any relaxing oil such as neroli, orange or rose oil can help, as a massage, added to the bath water or inhaled from a handkerchief or the pillow.

Nausea and vomiting

One of the earliest symptoms to alert a woman to possible pregnancy is often nausea, with or without vomiting. This is thought to be due to the hormones oestrogen and chorionic gonadotrophin affecting the blood sugar levels, but is sometimes exacerbated by tiredness, stress and an accompanying loss of appetite. Unfortunately, as sickness is usually a first trimester disorder, many of the essential oils that could be of use are contraindicated during the vital weeks of early fetal cell and organ formation; some mothers may also dislike being touched at this time, so will not wish to receive massage.

A great deal of research has been carried out on the use of acupressure to the Pericardium 6 (P6) point for nausea and vomiting during pregnancy, as well as postoperatively and for patients receiving chemotherapy (Dundee *et al.*, 1988; Hyde, 1989; Stannard, 1989; Barsoum *et al.*, 1990; Dundee and Yang, 1990; Price *et al.*, 1991; De Aloysio and Penacchioni, 1992; Evans *et al.*, 1993; Belluomini *et al.*, 1994). It would appear that acupressure wrist bands (popularly used for motion sickness) can be effective in a significant number of women, and this would be an inexpensive means of treating some clients. The bands cost approximately £7 a pair and are reusable, so it would not be a major expense for a maternity unit to keep a supply for loan.

Some women do not respond to these bands, and for those with true hyperemesis gravidarum it may be too late to use them. A question has also been raised by some midwives about their effects on intravenous lines sited in the dorsum of the hand, although personal experience of the author has not revealed any complications. However, it is certainly worth trying the bands if the mother will wear them (Fig. 7.11). To position the bands correctly, the length of the mother's inner forearm, from wrist crease to elbow, is divided into 12: this gives 12 Chinese anatomical inches. Measuring two anatomical inches up from the wrist crease, on the inner aspect between the two bones, will locate the mother's P6 point, against which the 'button' inside the wrist band should be pressed. Alternatively, the mother's fingers can be used to measure two and a half fingers width from the wrist crease, to determine the correct spot.

Reflexology could also be useful in treating gestational sickness.

Fig 7.11 Position of acupressure wrist bands to combat nausea and vomiting. Use mother's own fingers to locate P6 points—two and a half fingers width above wrist crease on inner aspect of arm: a slight dip will be felt when exact point is located.

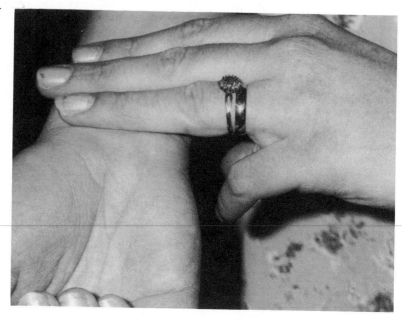

Table 7.5 Essential oils to combat nausea and vomiting

Camomile (not in early pregnancy)		Ginger	Grapefruit Lime
Mandarin Nutmeg (in labour)		Petitgrain	Sweet orange
Tangerine			

General relaxation techniques should be used together with work on the foot zones for the pituitary gland, hepatorenal and digestive systems.

When using essential oils it is important to avoid those classed as emmenagogic, which leaves very few suitable for treating gestational nausea and vomiting (Table 7.5). The best oils are mandarin, tangerine, sweet orange, lime and grapefruit (as long as the mother is not allergic to citrus fruit), all of which will assist in relaxing her, plus ginger to act as an antiemetic. Gentle massage of the back and shoulders, or, if the mother can cope with it, of the abdomen may help to ease both nausea and tension.

Grapefruit is thought to regulate appetite and act as a tonic for the biliary and hepatic systems, particularly in the digestion of fats, so it may be helpful in conjunction with dietary advice for women who are nauseated after eating food with a high fat content. Grapefruit is an especially refreshing essential oil; alternatively, the mother could be encouraged to eat grapefruit regularly during the day—grapefruit contains vitamin B$_6$ in which some women who suffer sickness may be deficient.

Ginger tea made from a piece of ginger root steeped in boiling water, with honey added to combat hypoglycaemia, can be sipped whenever the woman requires it. Although mothers should refrain from using essential oil of camomile in early pregnancy as it is emmenagogic, camomile tea can be drunk, perhaps with ginger root added to enhance the effects.

Price (1993, p.231) recommends petitgrain essential oil dropped on to the pillow to enable the woman to inhale the vapours overnight in preparation for the morning. She also suggests melissa tea made from the fresh herbs.

There appears to be confusion between different authorities over the use of peppermint essential oil, which is often cited as an effective antiemetic. Much research has been conducted into the toxicity of peppermint's menthol and pulegone content, the latter having been found to cause lesions in the brains of rats (Olsen and Thorup, 1984). Elder *et al.* (1960) found that menthol may have progesterone-like effects on liver enzymes, and, in view of the fact that no conclusions have yet been drawn, this author considers that peppermint should be avoided during early pregnancy, although it may be a valuable antiemetic to use well diluted during labour.

Labouring women often vomit due to raised adrenaline levels, stress and hypoglycaemia. Several antiemetic essential oils can be administered to make them feel refreshed and uplifted. Nutmeg oil in low proportions is antiemetic and is thought to have an oestrogenic action, thus strengthening contractions. A flask of hot camomile tea could be made in advance to deal with nausea if it arises, or ice cubes of camomile tea can be sucked throughout labour.

If a newborn baby vomits, the cause must obviously be sought, but in the early days it may be due to ingestion of mucous and fluid at delivery. Davis (1988, p. 71) suggests that one of the gentlest essential oils for children is camomile, which is effective as a relaxant, an antispasmodic in cases of colic and an antiemetic. The baby could be bathed in water to which a 1 per cent blend of camomile has been added, or receive an abdominal massage (clockwise) with the same blend. This is a non-invasive means of evacuating ingested amniotic fluid, rather than submitting the baby to a stomach wash-out. Alternatively, a teaspoon of camomile tea could be administered orally. Mandarin may have similar effects.

An unsuccessful case

Rosemary was admitted to the antenatal ward at six and a half weeks of pregnancy with 'hyperemesis gravidarum'—persistent nausea and vomiting two or three times a day. Conventional antiemetics failed to stop the vomiting and Rosemary seemed unable to eat anything without regurgitation, causing her to avoid eating.

She was given acupressure bands to wear on her wrists at the Pericardium 6 point. Camomile tea with the addition of honey and ginger root was suggested and she was advised to eat grapefruit. Rosemary declined reflexology at this time, preferring not to be 'messed about with'.

Three days after admission Rosemary required an intravenous infusion to replace lost fluid; the wrist bands had been left on but had been moved when the cannula was sited and, needless to say, Rosemary felt that they had been ineffective.

Over the next 2 weeks the complementary therapy midwife visited Rosemary several times to check on her progress and to offer reflexology and/or aromatherapy; finally, in desperation, she agreed to a foot massage incorporating reflexology and using some of the citrus essential oils. This certainly helped her to relax but Rosemary was still not eating and continued to vomit once or twice a day. The consultant decided to commence parenteral nutrition to provide vital nutrients, but agreed with the midwife that, when this was discontinued, homoeopathic remedies could be offered; these were also unsuccessful.

There did, however, appear to be psychological factors contributing to Rosemary's condition. She enjoyed the attention she received from the complementary therapist—to such an extent that eventually it was deemed to be detrimental to her recovery.

Rosemary went home after 3 weeks but, despite several readmissions, no real resolution of the sickness occurred until delivery.

Oedema

Oedema occurs in approximately 50 per cent of all pregnant women towards term, more commonly at the end of the day, and is sometimes worse in the first few days of the puerperium while the kidneys struggle to cope with autolysis and consequent increased diuresis as the mother's body returns to the non-pregnant state. Bimanual upwards massage of the ankles and lower legs will help to relieve excess fluid, and can be very relaxing. This could be demonstrated to the expectant mother by the midwife in the antenatal clinic, who could then ask someone at home to perform it for her. If the mother has bare legs, lubricant will be needed to avoid skin to skin friction, but this does not necessarily have to be a massage oil; talcum powder or soap and water are equally as

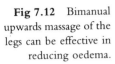

Fig 7.12 Bimanual upwards massage of the legs can be effective in reducing oedema.

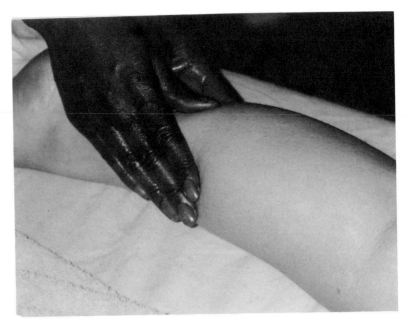

effective. If the mother is wearing tights, the massage can be carried out without any lubricant as the material will allow the hands to glide freely over the legs (Fig. 7.12).

Oedematous feet in the puerperium can cause the mother both physical and emotional distress, but some gentle massage of the dorsum of each foot, working from the toes towards the ankles, may disperse some of the fluid and give temporary relief. Likewise, finger oedema may be reduced by firm massage of each finger from the nail towards the hand and wrist, and, once demonstrated, the mother could do this for herself.

Shiatsu to the K2 point, on the middle of the arch of the foot, and K6, one thumb's width below the inside of the ankle bone (Fig. 7.13) can also be useful in alleviating ankle oedema, while a general reflexology treatment is relaxing and aids circulation, thereby indirectly easing the oedema.

Essential oils that stimulate the circulation, such as cypress, juniper berry, geranium, lemon, rosemary, patchouli, lavender or ginger, may help. Two of the most effective circulatory stimulants are onion and garlic, but use of the essential oils may be rejected on account of the odours, so these can be added to the diet.

For localized oedema, for example carpal tunnel syndrome, a compress of juniper berry and/or cypress oils combined with

Fig 7.13 Shiatsu
points for reducing
oedema.

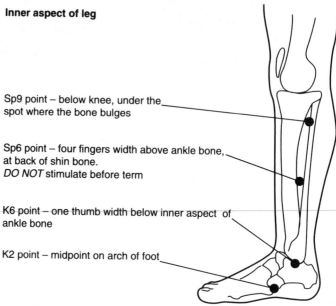

Inner aspect of leg

Sp9 point – below knee, under the
spot where the bone bulges

Sp6 point – four fingers width above ankle bone,
at back of shin bone.
DO NOT stimulate before term

K6 point – one thumb width below inner aspect of
ankle bone

K2 point – midpoint on arch of foot

Fig 7.14 Shiatsu
points to relieve carpal
tunnel syndrome.

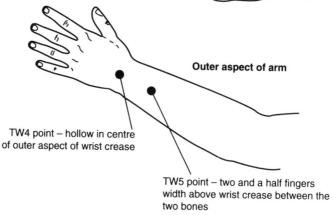

Outer aspect of arm

TW4 point – hollow in centre
of outer aspect of wrist crease

TW5 point – two and a half fingers
width above wrist crease between the
two bones

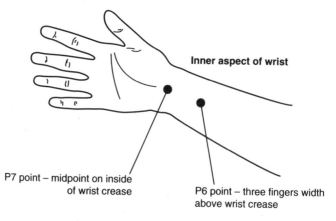

Inner aspect of wrist

P7 point – midpoint on inside
of wrist crease

P6 point – three fingers width
above wrist crease

exercise may reduce the intensity of the discomfort; shiatsu on the P6 and P7 points of the inner aspect of the forearm, and TW5 and TW4 on the corresponding parts of the outer arm can be self-administered (Fig. 7.14).

Pain relief in labour

Pain relief in labour may be obtained by using massage, with or without essential oils, especially gentle abdominal effleurage in a clockwise direction. This will serve to lessen the perception of pain as the touch impulses reach the brain before the pain impulses. Labouring women often appreciate neck and shoulder massage to loosen tense muscles. This may be accompanied by gradual pressure being applied to the GB21 shiatsu point on the shoulders (Fig. 7.9).

Foot massage with reflexology can be performed for relaxation and pain relief using brisk massage to the heels and stimulation of the pelvic lymphatic zones across the tops of the ankles (Fig. 7.15). The midwife can suggest that the mother carries out 'wrist wringing' (the equivalent pelvic lymphatic zones on the hands) for 5 minutes every hour to ease pelvic congestion (Fig. 7.16), together with acupressure to the LI4 point on the hand. Shiatsu to the points in the lumbosacral area (B27–B34) is simple and effective, and could be taught to partners (Fig. 7.9).

In labour, the range of essential oils that can be utilized is considerable (Table 7.6), but those selected for an individual will depend on the complete symptom picture. A mother who is very frightened and anxious, and whose perception of pain is therefore increased, may benefit from an oil that is a strong analgesic such as nutmeg or black pepper, combined with a calming oil (mandarin or lime) and a uterine toner in the form of rose. A primigravida having a long first stage due to an occipito-posterior position of the fetus could receive clary sage for pain, rose and lavender to stimulate contractions, together with camomile or geranium to relax her and to facilitate rest and sleep between contractions.

Midwives in Oxford carried out a 6-month trial using a variety of essential oils in labour, which included camomile, clary sage, eucalyptus, frankincense, jasmine, lavender, lemon, mandarin, peppermint and rose (Burns and Blamey, 1994). Most women and midwives found the use of aromatherapy in labour a pleasant and satisfying experience; the range of oils used enabled midwives to offer mothers a choice.

Nutmeg is advocated by some aromatherapists as it is not only analgesic but also calming and a circulatory stimulant; rose is thought

Fig 7.15
Reflexology to ease
contraction pains.

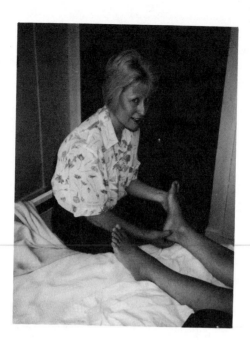

Fig 7.16 'Wrist
wringing' to ease
pelvic congestion in
labour.

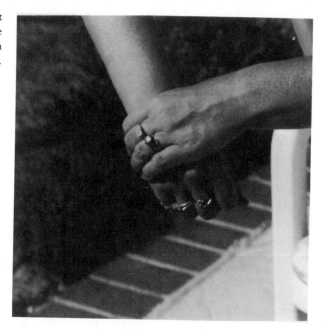

Table 7.6
Essential oils for the relief of pain in labour

Bergamot	Black pepper	Camomile	Clary sage	Eucalyptus
Frankincense	Geranium	Grapefruit	Jasmine	Lavender
Lemon	Lemongrass	Lime	Mandarin	Marjoram	Nutmeg
Peppermint	Petitgrain	Rose	Sandalwood	Tangerine
Ylang ylang				

to be a uterine relaxant with some analgesic action. Some oils act both as pain relievers and as a stimulant to the uterus, especially clary sage, jasmine, frankincense and rose, while others may be calming yet uplifting—mandarin, orange, bergamot and lemon. It is wise to be guided by the mother's choice of oils, as some may be cloying or nauseating, or she may simply dislike the aroma. The oils could be massaged into the feet, abdomen, shoulders and back, or they could be added to a bath or a foot bath. If vaporizers are available, the oils could be intermittently vaporized; compresses could be applied to the suprapubic or sacral areas; or a few drops of essential oil could be placed on a handkerchief.

Localized discomforts during labour may also occur, perhaps as a result of the mother's position. Massage to the shoulders with an oil such as orange, mandarin, lime or grapefruit can be relaxing and pleasant; foot massage with clary sage, frankincense or black pepper is warming; headache may be relieved by rubbing lavender and peppermint into the temples. If the mother is becoming emotionally stressed or very anxious, application of a calming oil such as ylang ylang directly to the solar plexus area beneath the xiphisternum, or to the related reflex zones on the feet, may help to calm her and to cope with the contractions, and the Bach flower remedy, Rescue Remedy, should be readily available.

Perineal care

Perineal massage towards term can be performed by the mother if she has a rigid perineum (such as in dancers and horse riders), or when a previous delivery has resulted in considerable scarring of the area. It assists in softening the tissues, increasing elasticity and facilitating the stretching that will occur during delivery. It may also help psychologically if the mother is unused to touching this part of her body, and may prepare her for midwifery interventions and care such as vaginal examinations.

The mother can be advised to perform the massage lying on her back in the bath. The thumb is inserted into the introitus with the first two fingers of the hand on the external perineal skin. A gentle massage can be performed, rubbing the thumb and fingers together in an upwards and outwards direction to stretch the perineum. It is not necessary to use any lubricant but if the mother prefers to do this on her bed she may need a little good-quality olive oil.

Some women like to continue perineal massage during labour, and occasionally incorporate clitoral massage which increases the production of endorphins, the brain's natural morphine-like analgesics, and can be very effective in reducing the woman's perception of contraction pain.

In the puerperium, perineal care revolves around easing discomfort, promoting healing and preventing infection. Dale and Cornwell's (1994) trial involved the use of essential oil of lavender in the bath, and although the results in relation to wound healing were not considered statistically significant there is some evidence that mothers experienced less perineal discomfort between the third and fifth postnatal day. Experience in the author's maternity unit supports this, and mothers have (anecdotally) been found to be more relaxed when using lavender in twice-daily baths for a number of days.

Lavender, having antibacterial properties, is effective in preventing infection, although if an episiotomy wound shows signs of infection the use of tea tree in the bidet is advocated. Camomile, eucalyptus or thyme may also be of use, while geranium or juniper berry oils aid healing, partly due to their astringent vasoconstrictive action.

Placenta, retained In women who have successfully completed the second stage of labour but in whom the placenta is slower than normal to separate, essential oils can be used to initiate uterine action. Jasmine oil, massaged over the fundus, lavender or clary sage can be used. It may, however, be easier and more effective for the midwife to perform reflexology on the foot zones relating to both the uterus and the pituitary gland to stimulate uterine contraction (Fig. 7.10).

A compress of basil or camomile oil applied suprapubically can relieve 'afterpains', aid involution and encourage any retained products to be expelled.

Preconception care and infertility

The midwife may not often come into contact with women who are planning to conceive, but she may be asked for information regarding the use of aromatherapy for subsequent pregnancies.

As with all drugs, essential oils should be used with caution during the preconception period and in the first trimester of pregnancy, and self-administration should perhaps be discouraged. Aromatherapy can be of value in relaxing couples whose desire to conceive is proving emotionally and physically stressful. Gentle oils such as orange, mandarin, grapefruit, frankincense and ylang ylang could be used in low dilutions for massage or in the bath. Culinary herbs could be added to the diet as a means of obtaining small amounts of the necessary essential oils.

Massage, reflexology or shiatsu relax either the prospective mother or father, and could then be continued into the pregnancy. Experience of this author and other reflex zone therapists in identifying, on the relevant foot zones, when and from which ovary ovulation has occurred, and in tracking the movement of the ovum along the fallopian tube, may indicate a potential use for reflexology in the treatment of infertility. It should theoretically be possible for stimulation of the foot zones related to the pituitary gland and the ovary to trigger ovulation.

Respiratory problems

It may appear to be a coincidence that pregnant women suffer from coughs, colds and sinus congestion, in much the same way as any non-pregnant person. In Oriental medicine, however, persistent coughs in particular may indicate weak Kidney meridian energy (Johnson, 1995, p. 134) and the midwife could refer the mother to a qualified shiatsu practitioner for rebalancing of energy throughout the body. Chronic sinus congestion may be eased by eliminating dairy produce from the diet, as it is known to increase mucus production.

Symptomatic relief can be obtained with aromatherapy. For infectious respiratory conditions such as colds and influenza, essential oils of tea tree, eucalyptus, benzoin, clary sage, frankincense or marjoram can be inhaled and will both ease congestion and loosen mucus and also act as an antibacterial agent. Lavender can be effective when the mother has an accompanying headache, but only during the last trimester. The oils can be massaged into the upper back, using effleurage and some percussion techniques to aid mucus drainage. Adding garlic to the diet will fight any infection, or teas made from basil or camomile can be suggested.

Reflex zone therapy to the thoracic and head zones on the feet may assist expectoration of mucus and relieve headache respectively. Acupressure to the B2, LI20 and St3 points can ease sinus congestion, headache, tired eyes and other cold symptoms (Fig. 7.17).

Fig 7.17 Shiatsu points for sinus congestion.

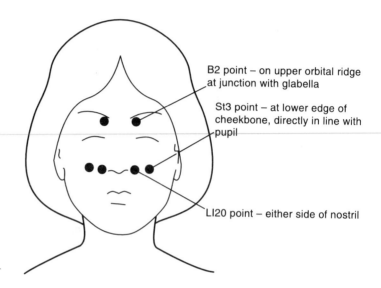

B2 point – on upper orbital ridge at junction with glabella

St3 point – at lower edge of cheekbone, directly in line with pupil

LI20 point – either side of nostril

Sexual difficulties Many expectant and newly delivered women experience a variety of emotional and physical symptoms which can adversely affect libido and physical comfort during sex. The more serious problems may require referral to an appropriate counsellor, but some difficulties can be resolved with aromatherapy.

Psychological and emotional factors may be helped by offering essential oil massages and/or baths using blends containing aphrodisiac ylang ylang, neroli and sandalwood during pregnancy, plus rose, patchouli, clary sage and jasmine in the puerperium. These may help to relax the woman (and her partner), and may work indirectly on the libido. Davis (1988, p. 33) suggests that black pepper and cardamom may have a directly stimulating effect and can be of use when fatigue is a predisposing factor, but they should be administered with caution only as a temporary measure (see Chapter 8).

If physical factors are contributing to sexual difficulties, the appropriate essential oils can be applied to deal with a sore perineum, thrush, leucorrhoea, etc.

Skin care   During the childbearing year some women find their skin becomes dehydrated, while others experience oiliness in the form of acne and skin eruptions. Many mothers develop striae gravidarum, usually as full term approaches. A few, especially brunettes and darker-skinned women, are bothered by excess melanin production, which results not only in pigmentation of the linea alba, but also facial chloasma. Aromatherapy has several remedies to offer for skin care; indeed, many people think that aromatherapy is only concerned with beauty care.

Dry skin may be helped by using gentle essential oils such as orange, neroli or rose in a base oil enriched with a small amount of avocado and wheatgerm oils. Apricot kernel or peach kernel are good base oils for facial massage. The mother can be advised to massage the oils into the skin very gently to avoid further damage. In early pregnancy the base oil can be used on its own. Davis (1988, p. 105) advocates the application of face packs containing honey and avocado or banana.

The high levels of circulating hormones can, in some women, have much the same effect as at the time of puberty, resulting in oily skin or even acne. Astringent and antibacterial essential oils are useful in these cases, including bergamot, cypress, lemon and sandalwood, and are best administered via a facial sauna rather than as a massage oil. Tea tree oil can be added to the blend if there are numerous spots; one drop can be applied neat to an isolated eruption, or a water-based spray can be applied over the whole area.

There is no evidence to indicate that application of any oil, lotion or cream can prevent striae gravidarum from developing, despite the plethora of proprietary products claiming to do so. If a mother wishes to apply aromatherapy oils to her abdomen to moisturize the outer skin, the most suitable are neroli and mandarin, possibly used in rotation with bergamot and rosewood. They can be applied after 16 weeks, in a base oil of soya, avocado and wheatgerm.

Chloasma, unfortunately, is unlikely to respond to treatment with aromatherapy oils, although Davis (1988, p. 203) states that lemon essential oil acts as a mild bleaching agent, as may benzoin. However, as daily use over a protracted period of time may be needed for the oil to take effect, the value of aromatherapy in reducing gestational chloasma is limited.

Eczema responds well to essential oils of lavender and camomile, and babies who develop the condition could be treated by adding two drops of essential oil to the bath water, using camomile for 1 week, lavender for 1 week with a 1-week interval between. It must be recognized, however, that in many cases this may treat the symptoms but not the cause of the eczema.

Stress and anxiety   Anxiety and stress are common during pregnancy and childbearing for a number of reasons, including fear of the unknown, concerns about the fetus/baby and lack of confidence. Obviously aromatherapy cannot take the place of sensitive midwifery care, talking and counselling. In many respects, however, this is one condition where aromatherapy comes into its own, and indeed is most likely to be perceived as acceptable by sceptical colleagues. There are several essential oils that can be used to combat stress (Table 7.7), although many are contraindicated during pregnancy. If there is any doubt regarding the safety of an essential oil, a simple massage—of feet, shoulders or back—using base oil alone is extremely relaxing.

Sedative and calming oils, including bergamot, benzoin, frankincense, geranium, mandarin, neroli, petitgrain, sandalwood and ylang ylang, are suitable for use in pregnancy. Other oils that can be administered near term, during labour or after delivery include camomile, clary sage, cypress, geranium, jasmine, juniper berry, lavender, marjoram, melissa, patchouli and rose.

There are a few other oils that are classified as sedative, such as cedarwood, celery, linden blossom, sage, verbena and vetivert, but these are not suitable for use in midwifery.

The most relaxing method of application may be in a massage, but adding a blend to the bath water or inhaling the aromas from a vaporizer will save time; respiratory tract administration is thought to have a direct effect upon the limbic system and on mood (Buchbauer *et al.*, 1991, 1993). If the anxiety is causing physical symptoms, oils can be selected specifically to relieve them. These would include (depending on the gestation) bergamot or marjoram for muscle tension, mandarin or neroli for stomach upsets, ylang ylang or lavender for raised blood pressure, lavender for headaches, and ylang ylang or camomile for insomnia. As a universal 'standby' which can be used from the second trimester in small doses, in labour, in the puerperium and for the neonate, the optimum

Table 7.7 Essential oils to combat stress

Benzoin	Bergamot	Camomile	Clary sage	Cypress
Frankincense	Geranium	Jasmine	Juniper berry	Lavender
Marjoram	Mandarin	Melissa	Neroli	Orange	Patchouli
Petitgrain	Rose	Sandalwood	Ylang ylang	

essential oil must be mandarin, particularly when given in a massage. However, administration should not be continuous for more than 3 weeks, and is best alternated with other oils to avoid allergy or irritation developing.

Urinary tract problems

Frequency of micturition is normally due to uterine pressure on the bladder and cannot be resolved with aromatherapy. However, essential oils could be used in the bidet as a vulval wash to prevent infection resulting from urethral contamination and the predisposing factor of urinary stasis. If infection occurs at any time during pregnancy or after delivery, bergamot and sandalwood can be applied as a suprapubic and sacral compress, or added to the bath or bidet. Drinking copious amounts of camomile tea will act as a urinary cleanser, and postnatally the essential oil can be used in the same way as bergamot and sandalwood. A 3 per cent synergistic blend of all three oils may be the most effective. Benzoin, frankincense and juniper berry oils also have strong antiseptic properties and can be used in the treatment of cystitis.

Where a mother suffers from retention of urine, reflex zone therapy offers a simple means of stimulating the urinary tract; indeed selected midwives could be taught the specific technique as part of their range of additional skills within the Scope of Professional Practice (UK Central Council, 1992a).

Sally had developed antenatal retention of urine at 16 weeks which, although not confirmed by ultrasound investigation, was deemed to be due to a retroverted gravid uterus. The complementary therapy midwife was asked to see her at 20 week's gestation, by which time Sally had a self-retaining catheter in situ (although she was still an outpatient). The midwife performed reflex zone therapy, and on examination was astounded to feel, on the relevant part of Sally's feet, that the zone for the uterus was further back on the heel than would normally be felt. This seemed to indicate that the assumed diagnosis of retroversion was correct.

The midwife carried out one full session of reflex zone therapy, after which Sally spontaneously passed 400 ml urine. One might consider that, at 20 weeks' gestation, the situation may have resolved itself anyway, but it is interesting that spontaneous micturition occurred shortly after the first treatment. The catheter was removed and was not needed again. Sally chose to continue to receive reflex zone therapy regularly and was able to enjoy her pregnancy to the full. Following a normal delivery of a large boy, she was unable to pass urine spontaneously for 18 hours, but reflex zone therapy was again successful.

Vaginal infections

As well as the normal physiological leucorrhoea that occurs in pregnancy, some women develop pruritus or vaginal infections such as candidiasis, *Trichomonas* or *Chlamydia*.

Sitting in a bath or washing the affected area with water to which has been added essential oils of bergamot, eucalyptus or frankincense may be effective in keeping the vulva free from infection when excessive leucorrhoea is a problem.

Where signs and symptoms of infection are present, the oil of choice is tea tree. Blackwell (1991) reported the effectiveness of tea tree pessaries in a woman with anaerobic vaginosis; Pena (1962) used it for *Trichomonas*; and the antimicrobial, antifungal, antiviral, antibacterial and antiseptic activities of tea tree have been extremely well documented (Belaiche, 1985a, 1985b; Shemesh and Mayo, 1991; Mayo, 1992; Carson and Riley, 1993, 1994; Kirwin, 1993; Emeny, 1994; Neilan, 1994).

Women can buy proprietary pessaries for self-administration if they suffer bouts of candidal infection during pregnancy; vulval washes containing tea tree would be helpful as a preventive measure post-caesarean section, or indeed simply after delivery if the lochia are heavy, in which case it could be added to the bath water.

Although genital herpes during pregnancy requires close medical supervision, tea tree essential oil can be added to the bath water to relieve itching and pain, and possibly to reduce the severity of the acute phase; Drury (1991) recommends 30 drops. Alternatively the oil can be applied neat to the herpes blisters to aid healing and prevent new eruptions. Tea tree is also effective in eliminating genital (and non-genital) warts: one drop of neat oil should be applied three times a day.

Varicosities

Varicose veins of the legs are usually temporary, developing in pregnancy as a result of the action of progesterone in relaxing the smooth walls of the blood vessels, and exacerbated by pressure from increasing abdominal weight. Complete resolution will not be achieved until after delivery, but essential oil of cypress in the bath water may assist in toning the circulation and reducing the throbbing pain that often accompanies varicose veins. Massage directly over varicosed areas is contraindicated, but gently gliding the hands over the leg will give an impression of 'completeness', especially during a full-body massage.

Similarly, if a mother suffers from vulval varicosities, cypress, juniper berry or lavender oil added to a bidet are astringent and help to soothe the discomfort.

Chapter 8

Directory of Oils for Use in

Midwifery Practice

Comprehensive information about individual essential oils can be found in many aromatherapy textbooks, and midwives are referred to the list of further reading in the References section for those recommended by the author, although this list is by no means exhaustive.

However, for ease of learning for midwives new to the subject of aromatherapy, a selection of essential oils suitable for use with pregnant, labouring and puerperal women and their newborn babies is included here, with emphasis on aspects of particular relevance to the client group. There is some repetition between this chapter and the previous one, but this should enable a cross-referencing system to be used, so that midwives can either refer to a specific essential oil or find information on oils most suited to the treatment of different conditions.

Each essential oil is identified by its Latin name; the main chemical constituents, and the uses and contraindications or dangers pertinent to midwifery practice are discussed.

The 30 essential oils outlined here are:

- Basil
- Benzoin
- Bergamot
- Black pepper

- Camomile
- Clary sage
- Eucalyptus
- Frankincense

- Geranium
- Ginger
- Grapefruit
- Jasmine
- Juniper berry
- Lavender
- Lemon
- Lemongrass
- Lime
- Mandarin
- Marjoram

- Neroli
- Nutmeg
- Orange
- Patchouli
- Petitgrain
- Rose
- Rosemary
- Rosewood
- Sandalwood
- Tea tree
- Ylang ylang

Basil—
Ocimum basilicum
(Labiatae family)

There are many different types of basil oil available but the one normally used in aromatherapy has a spicy aroma, derived by steam distillation from the flowers and leaves.

Chemical constituents Basil oil is very stimulating, even in small doses, due to the proportion of esters (about 8 per cent according to Price, 1993, p.54) and the monoterpenes limonene and pinene. The presence of the ketone, camphor, not only adds to the stimulant effect but is also an emmenagogue so basil is *contraindicated in pregnancy*. However, the monoterpenes, ketones and a high level of phenols means that basil has analgesic properties and can be of help in low dilutions in labour and the puerperium.

The amount of phenols is reputed to be as high as 40–50 per cent (Davis, 1988, pp. 49–50), which makes the essential oil an effective antiseptic. These, together with the alcohols, fenchol, linalol and citronellol and the oxide 1.8 cineole, have decongestant and expectorant effects so that basil can be used for inhalations in the event of chest infection, perhaps after a Caesarean section. Women who suffer respiratory tract congestion and sinus problems in pregnancy could make basil tea from the leaves, thus ensuring a weaker solution, and inhale the vapours. The antifungal properties of *Ocimum basilicum* have also been demonstrated (Dube *et al.*, 1989).

Basil is effective for headache and migraine, although there are other, safer oils which can be used in pregnancy for this complaint.

The antispasmodic action of basil as a result of the esters and phenols make it a useful oil for digestive complaints. The oestrogenic effects mean that it can aid placental separation in the third stage of labour and ease 'after pains' and breast engorgement in the early puerperium, as well as helping in cases of dysmenorrhoea and the menopause. It is thought to have a possible value in treating hormonally related infertility. Indeed, the stimulation of blood flow and the hormonal influence of basil, coupled with the effect on mental fatigue, make this a suitable oil to combine with others for massage in the early postnatal days.

Dangers   Basil is *contraindicated in pregnancy* because it is a stimulant and an emmenagogue. The high proportion of phenols, particularly methyl chavicol, can cause skin irritation to those with sensitive skin; there has also been speculation about potential carcinogenic effects of basil. High concentrations can reverse the generally stimulating effect and cause the recipient to become soporific.

Blends   Basil will blend well with bergamot, black pepper, clary sage, frankincense, geranium, grapefruit, lavender, lemongrass, mandarin, marjoram, neroli, rosemary, sandalwood and tangerine.

Benzoin—
Styrax benzoin
(Styracea family)

Benzoin comes from the eastern areas of Thailand and Java, and the resin is obtained from the bark of the tree. Solvent extraction (often with wood alcohol) is used to release the aromatic material from the resin. The aroma is pleasant and rather like vanilla.

Chemical constituents   Benzoin has an impact on the kidneys, stimulating renal output and, with its antiseptic property resulting from the aldehydes benzoic aldehyde and vanillin (which give it the characteristic aroma), may be of use in cystitis. Aldehydes can also be hypotensive in action. It is useful for treating colic, flatulence and constipation (in the mother), due to the antispasmodic action of the ester benzyl benzoate, and may help to control blood sugar levels (Sellar, 1992, p. 15).

Although benzoin is uplifting and stimulating, it is not an emmenagogue, so unlike basil could safely be used in low dilutions from mid-pregnancy, although the therapeutic effects of benzoin can be found in other oils which have been more frequently used on pregnant women. Its action on the respiratory tract, particularly in stimulating mucus flow, results in benzoin being useful as an inhalation for sinusitis, bronchitis, colds and coughs, and sore throats.

Benzoin is popularly known as Friar's Balsam for healing skin wounds, especially where there is dermatitis. It is possible that chloasma may be reduced if benzoin is added to a skin toner. The wound-healing and anti-inflammatory effects are probably due to the presence of acids—benzoic and cinnamic. However, cases of sensitivity to benzoin dressings have been reported (Cullen *et al.*, 1974; Mann, 1982; James *et al.*, 1984; Rademaker and Kirby, 1987; Tripathi *et al.*, 1990; Lesesne, 1992).

Stress, tension and anxiety can be calmed by using benzoin in a massage blend as it has a sedative effect and assists in easing worries and improving self-confidence; this may be of help in the postnatal period for some mothers.

Dangers If used to excess benzoin may cause drowsiness; in some people it may also cause allergic skin reactions (see above).

Blends Benzoin can be blended with bergamot, camomile, eucalyptus, frankincense, juniper berry, lavender, lemon, mandarin, orange, neroli, petitgrain, rose and sandalwood.

Bergamot—
Citrus bergamia
(Rutacea family)

Essential oil of bergamot is obtained by expression of the rind of the fruit from the tree, which is native to Italy. The aroma is mainly orange and lemon, and the oil is emerald green in colour.

Chemical constituents The proportion of alcohols, including linalol, nerol and geraniol, and the aldehyde citral means that bergamot has antiseptic properties coupled with an affinity for the urogenital tract, and provides a safe and effective means of treating cystitis and urinary tract infection throughout the reproductive year. It can relieve gastrointestinal complaints for which an antispasmodic is needed such as indigestion, colic and flatulence, as there are up to 50 per cent esters (Ryman, 1991, p. 53), including linalyl acetate, in bergamot oil. It is also thought to stimulate the appetite.

Monoterpenes (limonene, pinene and camphene), as well as the esters give bergamot its antiseptic, antibacterial, antiviral and antifungal characteristics. Respiratory tract infections respond well to inhalations of bergamot oil, as do certain viral infections such as herpes simplex and varicella. This is also due to the large amount of the aldehyde citral. Women who suffer from acne during pregnancy may find a facial sauna using bergamot will help to alleviate the condition. Citral is also responsible for acting as a hypotensive agent, as are the coumarins, mainly in the form of bergaptene. In addition, coumarins can have an anticoagulant effect and, although the proportion of these is small, it may be wise to use low dilutions towards term when the mother's own clotting mechanisms adapt to the impending labour.

Bergamot may help to tone the uterus and can be a good oil to use in labour, especially as it is also a very calming yet uplifting oil, possibly owing to its action on the sympathetic nervous system. It is antispasmodic and anti-inflammatory due to the presence of esters, while camphene, limonene and pinene (terpenes) are analgesic.

Dangers   The presence of a 0.44 per cent concentration of the furocoumarins bergaptene and bergamotine, which stimulate melanin production, means that this essential oil should be used with care. This is particularly important when there is bright sunlight, for excessive and irregular discoloration of exposed skin can occur; these areas of the body may possibly degenerate at a later stage and lead to early skin cancer. Reported cases in the 1970s (Meyer, 1970) of skin reactions to tanning agents containing bergamot, severe enough to require admission to a burns unit, eventually led to the oil being omitted from suntanning creams and lotions. Ryman (1991, p. 54) suggests that it should rarely be used as a massage oil, although other authorities state that it may be used in a 1–2 per cent dilution (International School of Aromatherapy, 1993, p. 75), while Price (1993, p. 54) argues that it is fully absorbed into the bloodstream within an hour, after which time the phototoxicity is negated. However, the raised melanocytic hormone levels during pregnancy emphasize the need for caution when using bergamot, as irregular patches of pigmentation may develop if the skin is exposed to the sun immediately after using high dilutions of the oil.

In addition the high citral content could potentially impair reproductive performance (Toaff et al., 1979; see Part 1).

Blends   Bergamot essential oil has a gentle aroma which blends well with basil, benzoin, black pepper, camomile, clary sage, eucalyptus, geranium, grapefruit, jasmine, juniper berry, lavender, lemon, mandarin, marjoram, neroli, orange, patchouli, petitgrain, rose, tangerine and ylang ylang.

Black pepper—
Piper nigrum
(Piperaceae
family)

Essential oil of black pepper is distilled from the fruit and seeds of the tree and, as might be expected, has a spicy peppery aroma, which appeals to men but which can also add interest to a more feminine blend (Plate 3).

Chemical constituents   The high concentration of monoterpenes (camphene, farnesene, limonene, myrcene, pinene, sabinene and thujene) and sesquiterpenes (caryophyllene) makes black pepper an excellent analgesic, and its vasodilatory effects make it valuable in cases of muscular aches, pains and stiffness. It is beneficial both before and after strenuous physical activity, and lends itself to pain relief in labour; it is also stimulating and seems to give mental stamina which could help a woman having a long, slow first stage.

Alcohols in the form of linalol and pinocarvol give black pepper a warming action which improves the circulation, making it beneficial for bruising. The oil could be applied postnatally in a massage to the buttocks where forceps delivery has resulted in excessive trauma. Despite its rubefacient characteristic, black pepper can also be used in small doses, almost in a homoeopathic way, to reduce pyrexia. The essential oil may increase the production of red blood cells, which could be valuable in cases of anaemia.

Black pepper contains phenols—carvocrol, eugenol, safrole and myristicin—which affect the digestive system. Its laxative properties make it a useful aid to increasing peristalsis and reducing flatulence. It is thought to help the digestion of proteins and the excretion of toxins, leading to weight loss, so it may appeal to women for use towards the end of the puerperium. The oil has strong diuretic properties but should not be used directly for this purpose as overdosing could precipitate excessive renal stimulation; low doses are advised during pregnancy to avoid potential damage to kidney function.

Dangers   The above-mentioned diuretic effect needs to be taken into consideration when using black pepper in pregnancy. Very small amounts can be beneficial but care should be taken that it is blended with other oils to reduce the concentration. It is also possible that higher concentrations may lead to skin irritation, so vaporization rather than massage may be the preferred method of administration. Ryman (1991, p. 159) comments on its myristicin content, which, although much lower than the amount in nutmeg or mace oils, may be sufficient to preclude its use during pregnancy (see also Nutmeg).

Blends Small amounts of black pepper give a blend an interesting spiciness and it mixes well with basil, bergamot, frankincense, geranium, grapefruit, lemon, mandarin, nutmeg, patchouli, rosemary, sandalwood and ylang ylang.

Camomiles—
Matricaria
chamomilla and
Anthemis nobilis
(Compositae
family)

There are several different types of camomile essential oil available, each with slightly different, though mainly similar, properties. The commonest camomiles used in aromatherapy are German camomile, *Matricaria chamomilla*, and the purer and more expensive Roman camomile, *Anthemis nobilis*. A Moroccan variety, *Ormenis multicaulis*, is also sometimes used. All camomiles belong to the Compositae family, but it is important to obtain the essential oil from a reputable supplier and to ask for it by its Latin name as the proportion of the chemical constituents varies from one type to another. (This is similar to the need to ask for drugs by their trade name rather than the generic name to ensure the exact composition.)

The two most commonly used camomile essential oils will be considered here: German and Roman camomiles.

Matricaria chamomilla Despite its name, the plant is no longer grown in Germany for essential oil production, but comes mainly from eastern Europe, particularly Hungary. The essential oil is distilled from the flowers and initially is a bluish colour which gradually alters to a greenish yellow colour. The depth of the blue coloration is dependent on the amount of chamazulene, a constituent that is not present in the flower but develops during the process of extracting the essential oil, and German camomile tends to be deeper blue than Roman as it contains more chamazulene. It is interesting to note that the term *Matricaria* comes from the Latin meaning uterus, and indeed camomile has a long history in folk medicine of being used for gynaecological problems.

Chemical constituents The presence of the sesquiterpene, azulene, a fatty substance which forms during the production process, results in German camomile's anti-inflammatory and wound-healing properties; it is especially effective in treating skin problems such as eczema. This and another sesquiterpene, farnesene, together with the alcohols, farnesol and bisabolol, and the aldehyde, cuminic acid, also contribute to the antiseptic, antibacterial, antifungal and antiviral functions of camomile; Ryman (1991, p. 77) states that camomile may be 120 times more effective than saline in acting as an antiseptic.

Camomile seems to have a particular affinity for the urinary tract, so women with a urinary tract infection or cystitis could drink camomile tea as a urinary cleanser. Using a dilute solution of the tea as an eye cleanser may prevent or treat ophthalmia neonatorum.

Soaked and cooled camomile teabags placed over sore and bleeding nipples can ease discomfort and speed healing, without danger to the infant of accidentally ingesting a harmful substance which might otherwise be applied to heal the nipples. However, two mothers are reported to have developed contact dermatitis of the nipple after applying Kamillosan cream, a popular cream containing essential oil of camomile (McGeorge and Steele, 1991). Interestingly, one mother was using a British brand of Kamillosan which contains Roman camomile while the other, in Europe, was using a brand containing German camomile. On the other hand the wound-healing, anti-inflammatory and analgesic properties of *M. chamomilla* have been well documented (Tubaro *et al.*, 1984; Aertgeerts *et al.*, 1985; Glowania *et al.*, 1987; Nissen *et al.*, 1988). It can safely be surmised that sitting in a bath to which camomile oil has been added may assist in healing the perineum following delivery, and will help to relax the mother.

Recent research (Safayhi *et al.*, 1994) suggests that the antiphlogistic effects of camomile may be due to the inhibition by chamazulene of the production of leucotrienes, found in patients with various inflammatory diseases.

A small amount of camphor, which is a ketone, means that camomile is an emmenagogue, so use of the essential oil should be *avoided in early pregnancy*, although judicious use in later pregnancy is acceptable and the beneficial effects of camomile's constituents can be obtained by drinking the tea during the first and second trimesters.

Ketones and sesquiterpenes make camomile a good analgesic: teabags placed against the neck over the eustachian tube can ease earache; the essential oil massaged into the back relieves backache, dysmenorrhoea or the pain of contractions and afterpains; headaches may also be helped by using camomile.

Anthemis nobilis Although there are many similarities in the therapeutic properties of *A. nobilis* and *M. chamomilla*, the plants are very different, with *A. nobilis* being shorter, the stems hairier and the white daisy-like flowers larger than those of *M. chamomilla*.

Chemical constituents As with German camomile, the essential oil of *A. nobilis* contains chamazulene (sesquiterpene) and cuminic acid (aldehyde), which make it antiseptic, antibacterial, antiviral and antifungal, as well as pain relieving. Other monoterpenes, such as camphene, myrcene and pinene, plus sesquiterpenes (β-caryopllyl-lene and sabinene) increase the analgesic effects.

There is a very high proportion of esters such as angelic acid, tiglic acid and methacrylic acid, which may be between 50 per cent (Price, 1993, p. 54) and 85 per cent (Lawless, 1992, p. 80). These not only add to the anti-infective effects but are also antispasmodic and relaxing. Roman camomile can be used as a relaxing massage oil in labour and will work on the digestive system to treat flatulence, heartburn, nausea and vomiting. However, due to the amount of the ketone pinocarvone (greater than the proportion of camphor in German camomile), *A. nobilis* essential oil has emmenagogic proper-ties and *should not be used in pregnancy* until almost term. The ketones and a small amount of coumarins have anticoagulant effects, and *A. nobilis* may also stimulate both the immune system and the produc-tion of blood constituents: leucocytes to fight infection and ery-throcytes to prevent anaemia.

There are small amounts of mono-alcohol in the form of bisabolol and farnesol in Roman camomile, which add to the anti-infective properties, as well as being vasoconstrictive which makes camomile a very warming oil. Conversely, in oils produced from crops in which the proportion of sesquiterpenes such as pinocarvol is greater, there may be an antipyretic as well as a hypotensive effect. Camomile generally is a very calming and gentle oil which can safely be used on children to help them sleep.

Dangers Camomile has emmenagogic effects so is *contraindicated in early pregnancy*, and, as noted above, Roman camomile should be avoided until almost term, although Tisserand and Balacs (1995, p. 111) dispute this, suggesting that it is safe to use throughout the gestational period. Contrary to its beneficial action on the skin, a few people may develop dermatitis from prolonged use of the essential oil, as in the case of a florist who was constantly handling the plants (Van Ketel, 1987). There has been a report of anaphylactic shock from camomile tea (cited by International School of Aromatherapy, 1993, p. 67), and it is possible that people sensitive to camomile pollen may develop allergic rhinitis.

Blends Either *M. chamomilla* or *A. nobilis* will blend well with benzoin, bergamot, clary sage, geranium, grapefruit, jasmine, lavender, lemon, mandarin, marjoram, neroli, orange, patchouli, rose, tangerine and ylang ylang.

Clary sage—
Salvia sclarea
(Labiatae family)

The white or blue flowers of this herb, grown in Europe and parts of America, provide the essential oil, which is extracted by steam distillation (Plate 1). The aroma is a rather heavy herbal smell, sometimes described as 'nutty'. It is important not to confuse clary sage with the more popularly known sage (Plate 2) for in aromatherapy the essential oil of sage should be used only by experienced practitioners. This is particularly significant in midwifery as there have been incidents of sage causing severe intermenstrual bleeding, menorrhagia and miscarriage.

Chemical constituents Due to the presence of the ester linalyl acetate, clary sage is anti-infective and acts as an uplifting nerve tonic. The alcohols linalol and sclareol are also present, adding to the antifungal, antiviral and antibacterial properties of the oil. The presence of the oxide 1.8 cineole makes clary sage a useful oil in cases of respiratory infection and congestion, for oxides are both expectorant and mucolytic; simply inhaling clary on a tissue can clear the nasal passages when one has a cold. However, the 1.8 cineole may also irritate the skin in sensitive people, so the oil should be well diluted for massage or in the bath.

The sesquiterpene caryophyllene gives clary essential oil analgesic and antispasmodic actions, so it is good for labour. Clary sage also seems to work well for premenstrual tension, dysmenorrhoea and 'after pains'. It may help with stress–related sexual problems. Unlike sage (*Salvia officinalis*), clary contains no ketones—it is the high proportion of thujone in sage which makes it an effective abortifacient and, according to Ryman (1991, p. 192) the level of thujone can be as much as 60 per cent in the sage oil obtained from Dalmatia.

Traces of the monoterpenes myrcene, phellandrene and pinene enhance the analgesic, anti-infective and expectorant properties of the oil and act as a stimulant, but may also exacerbate any potential skin irritation. Clary sage is certainly useful for its uplifting qualitites in both labour and the postnatal period, although large doses may have the reverse effect.

Dangers As mentioned above, large doses of clary sage may cause headaches or drowsiness: care should be taken over the timing of administration and women should be advised not to drive immediately afterwards. Clary is known to potentiate the effects of alcohol, so should not be used shortly before or after alcohol consumption. Although clary does not contain abortifacient ketones, it is thought to be emmenagogic and therefore *should be used with caution in pregnancy* until near term.

Blends Clary sage blends well with basil, bergamot, cedarwood, cypress, frankincense, geranium, grapefruit, jasmine, juniper berry, lavender, lime, mandarin, orange, patchouli, rose, tangerine and sandalwood.

Eucalyptus— *Eucalyptus globulus* (Myrtaceae family)

There are many different types of eucalyptus oil available, some such as *Eucalyptus radiata* having a camphorous aroma, others like *E. citriodora* possessing a citrussy aroma. The commonest type used is *E. globulus*, originally from Australia, although new varieties are being produced continually.

Chemical constituents The largest proportion of any chemical in eucalyptus oil is the oxide 1.8 cineole (possibly up to 80 per cent), making it a powerful expectorant and mucolytic but also a potential skin irritant. The alcohol globulol may be responsible for the oil's effectiveness in reducing pyrexia, while the monoterpenes camphene, fenchene, phellandrene and pinene, and the aldehyde citronellal, are antibacterial and antiviral. Consequently eucalyptus essential oil is valuable in respiratory tract infections and sinus congestion.

Tests on the antimicrobial activity of several different types of eucalyptus have shown very positive results (Hmamouch et al., 1990; Penoel, 1992; Gundidza et al., 1993; Hajji and Fkih-Tetouani 1993; Zakarya et al., 1993).

It is thought that there are over 250 constituents of eucalyptus oil (Ryman, 1991, p. 97), including various aldehydes, terpenes and sesquiterpenic alcohols, so it is difficult to attribute the various properties to specific constituents. However, eucalyptus has also been found to be useful for urinary tract infections due to its anti-infective and diuretic effects. Adding a small amount of the oil to bath water, deep enough to cover the suprapubic area could be helpful for women who develop cystitis in pregnancy. Sellar (1992, p. 57) suggests that it may be of use in cases of nephritis.

Dangers Eucalyptus is a strong essential oil, so only small doses should be used. Ingestion may lead to vomiting, central nervous system depression (Spoerke *et al.*, 1989) and even death (Leung, cited by Lawless, 1992, p. 94); in recounting the case of a small boy who ingested 10 ml of the oil, Patel and Wiggins (1980) quote the safe adult internal dosage as between 0.06 and 0.2 ml. Hypertensive women and epileptics (Sellar, 1992, p. 57) should avoid it; use in pregnancy appears to be acceptable (Pages *et al.*, 1990), although in this latter trial the authors recognize the need for further work on the teratogenic effects.

The strong aroma of eucalyptus oil may antidote homoeopathic remedies, 'so the two should not be stored together, nor should anyone using homoeopathy receive simultaneous eucalyptus.

Spoerke *et al.*'s work in 1989 described 14 cases of exposure to eucalyptus essential oil. Some skin irritation occurred but subsided within 1 hour; however, it would be wise to be aware of the possible effects on the skin when using this oil.

Blends Eucalyptus has an aroma that is familiar to most people and blends well with essential oils which subdue the intensity of the odour, such as benzoin, bergamot, ginger, juniper berry, lavender, lemon, melissa, tea tree and thyme.

Frankincense— Boswellia carteri (Burseraceae family) With its biblical associations it is evident that frankincense has been used for many centuries as an aromatic substance in the Church as well as for perfume and, indeed, medicinally. Oleo gum resin is extracted from the bark of the tree and the essential oil is obtained through steam distillation, although an absolute is also produced for use in the perfume industry. It may be more popularly known to some readers as olibanum, a proprietary product of which is available as a decongestant. It has a camphorous aroma, as one might expect, yet is fairly light and sweet.

Chemical constituents Frankincense contains mainly monoterpenes in the form of cymene, pinene, limonene, camphene, myrcene, thujene, phellandrene and dipentene, as well as some alcohols such as farnesol, borneol, octanol, olibanol and incensol. Together these chemicals make the essential oil a strong antiseptic, which is especially good as a room purifier, and is also antibacterial, antifungal and antiviral. The antimicrobial activity of directly distilled oil has been found to be effective against some organisms such as *Staphylococcus aureus* and *Escherichia coli* but not against *Pseudomonas aeruginosa* or *Candida albicans* (Abdel Wahab *et al.*, 1987).

The monoterpenes and the alcohols are, in addition, known to be decongestant and expectorant, so the oil is very useful as an inhalation or as part of a blend for chest and back massage, for respiratory tract infections, and helps to clear the head in cases of influenza and colds.

Frankincense is reported as having an affinity with the genitourinary tract (Lawless, 1992; Sellar, 1992; Tisserand, 1992) and can be used in the bath for women with cystitis, leucorrhoea and, in the non-pregnant woman, for dysmenorrhoea and metrorrhagia.

Frankincense is also thought to be an emmenagogue, although almost all authorities state that it is safe to use in pregnancy. Professional caution should be exercised, however, and it would be wise to use the oil only in the last trimester of pregnancy. In labour it can safely be used as a soothing massage oil, and postnatally may be helpful for women with depression. The presence of the alcohols means that the oil also has some vasoconstrictive effects, so making it a possible oil to use in cases of uterine haemorrhage, although this has not been demonstrated in midwifery practice.

Dangers Frankincense is generally considered to be a safe essential oil in all respects but, until more research is available about its emmenagogic effects, it is advisable during pregnancy to use it only in the last trimester.

Blends Frankincense is classed as a base note, in that its aroma is not immediately noticeable in a blend, but will linger for several hours; obviously the therapeutic effects continue to take place during this prolonged period of time. It will blend well with basil, benzoin, bergamot, black pepper, cedarwood, cinnamon, clary sage, geranium, ginger, grapefruit, jasmine, juniper berry, lavender, lemon, mandarin, melissa, myrrh, nutmeg, orange, patchouli, rosemary, rosewood, sandalwood and tangerine.

Geranium— Pelargonium graveolens or odorantissimum (Geraniaceae family)

Essential oil of geranium is distilled from the flowers of the shrub (Plate 4) to produce an oil with a rather heavy odour which may be similar to rose (*Pelargonium graveolens*) or somewhat apple-like (*P. odorantissimum*). The main producer of geranium oil is the island of Reunion, formerly known as Bourbon, and the best oil is still Bourbon geranium, although other countries are beginning to compete for production.

Chemical constituents Geranium oil has very strong anti-infective properties. The presence of alcohols such as terpenic geraniol, linalol, citronellol, borneol, myrtenol and terpineol mean that geranium is antibacterial, antifungal and antiviral. The aldehyde citral and the esters geranyl acetate, linalyl acetate, citronellyl acetate, valerianic acid and acetic acid enhance these properties.

The alcohols also give the oil stimulating and uplifting qualities, although the aldehyde may have the opposite effect. In some respects geranium seems to act rather like alcohol, in exacerbating the current mood of the recipient. Too high a proportion in a blend can also lead to either hyperactivity or to a heavy soporific feeling, so care should be taken to regulate the dose.

The alcohols are thought to be vasoconstrictors, which could lead to increased blood pressure, although the relaxing effects of the aldehydes through directly working on the adrenal cortex, and of the sesquiterpenes, would appear to counteract this. In the main geranium is used as a balancer and toner, acting particularly on the reproductive and urinary tracts.

The phenol, eugenol, may induce diuresis in women with inadequate elimination processes in whom the system is congested, and geranium can be helpful in reducing oedema and toning the liver, kidneys and general circulation. The alcohols also have some effect on the liver.

A combination of terpenes such as sabinene, limonene, β-caryophyllene and phellandrene, and of eugenol (phenol), with their analgesic properties, together with the anti-inflammatory effects of geranic acid result in geranium being a useful oil for both labour and the puerperium. The oil can be blended with lavender to ease the pain of contractions during labour, although the mother should be consulted about the aroma, as a blend of these two alone may be too cloying or nauseating for some. It could be added to bidets and baths for perineal care postnatally as it improves the circulation, and geranium leaves have been found to be useful for sore nipples (Minchin, 1994); conversely, vascular dermatitis from Bourbon geranium leaves has also been reported (International School of Aromatherapy, 1993, p. 74).

Dangers True geranium is expensive and it is possible to find cheaper brands of the oil which may have been adulterated with other essential oils such as lemongrass or cedarwood or with artificial esters (Ryman, 1991, p. 106). This is important for midwives, as cedarwood not only may be a skin irritant but is also thought to be both emmenagogic and abortifacient. Consequently care should be taken when purchasing geranium to ensure its purity.

Blends Geranium can be a very pleasant addition to many blends but is probably best used well diluted. It blends especially well with basil, bergamot, clary sage, grapefruit, jasmine, lavender, lemongrass, neroli, orange, petitgrain, rose, rosemary and sandalwood.

Ginger—
Zingiber officinale
(Zingiberaceae family)

As might be expected, ginger essential oil has a spicy, sharp, slightly woody aroma, with Jamaican ginger reputedly having the best smell. The oil is steam distilled from the dried ground root. Ginger has a very long history of medicinal use for stomach and digestive complaints in various cultures around the world.

Chemical constituents The sesquiterpene, zingiberene, and monoterpenes, camphene, limonene and *d*-phellandrene, make ginger an effective analgesic, particularly when combined with the warming effects of the alcohols, borneol and linalol, and the oxide 1.8 cineole. Ginger also has antiseptic and anti-infective characteristics due to the aldehyde citral, the alcohols and the monoterpenes.

The carminative and digestive actions of ginger appear to arise from the presence of the 1.8 cineole and the influence on the hepatic system of the alcohols. Ginger, in either essential oil or tea form, has long been used to stimulate gastric secretions and to treat flatulence, loss of appetite, diarrhoea, and nausea and vomiting. This makes the oil valuable for pregnancy—or the mother could be advised to drink the tea or chew crystallized ginger to combat nausea. The antiemetic effects have been documented and many midwives already inform mothers about its value (Roach, 1985).

Dangers Ginger oil is thought to have some low-level phototoxicity which is not significant when the oil is blended with non-phototoxic oils but may be exacerbated if mixed with phototoxic oils such as those from citrus plants. Sensitive people may develop skin irritation when the essential oil is applied in a massage blend.

Blends Ginger will blend well with eucalyptus, frankincense, geranium, lemon, lime, orange and rosemary, with the proviso to be cautious in women with skin sensitivity.

Grapefruit—
Citrus paradisi
(Rutaceae family)

This is a lovely refreshing essence which, together with other citrus oils, lends itself especially to pregnancy and childbearing. The essence is extracted by expression of the peel of the fruit but, as the yield is less than that of orange trees, grapefruit may be slightly more expensive.

Chemical constituents Grapefruit essence contains about 90 per cent of the monoterpene limonene, according to Lawless (1992, p. 105), which gives it strong antiseptic and analgesic properties. The 0.0012 per cent concentration of furocoumarins as a result of the process of extraction means that it has some phototoxic effects, although not as much as bergamot or lime (International School of Aromatherapy, 1993, p. 75), and the effect can be eliminated or 'quenched' if it is blended with other non-phototoxic oils (Price, 1993, p. 37), although Henson (personal communication, 1995) disputes this. It is also the furocoumarins which give the oil its calming yet refreshing effects. A 2 per cent blend of grapefruit provides a pleasant oil for a facial or gentle abdominal massage in pregnancy.

The presence of the aldehydes citral, citronellal and neral, although in small amounts, enhance the aroma of the essence and result in the anti-inflammatory, tonic, hypotensive and depurative properties. In addition, the small quantity of geraniol, a monoterpenol (alcohol), adds to the antibacterial and antiviral effects of grapefruit.

Grapefruit oil has a short shelf-life of about 3 months, so should be bought in small amounts, preferably stored in the refrigerator, blended only in the quantity required and discarded after the expiry date. Antioxidant (about 0.002 per cent) is often added to the essence to prevent premature deterioration (Price, 1993, p. 89).

Dangers As with other citrus oils there is some concern regarding the phototoxicity of grapefruit, although it appears to be less severe than that of bergamot. Grapefruit should be avoided if the client is allergic to citrus fruit, otherwise it is, as far as is known, a safe and pleasant essence to use intermittently throughout pregnancy.

Blends Grapefruit oil blends well with basil, bergamot, black pepper, camomile, clary sage, frankincense, geranium, jasmine, juniper berry, lavender, lemon, lemongrass, lime, mandarin, neroli, orange, tangerine, rose, rosemary, rosewood and ylang ylang.

Jasmine— **Jasminum** **officinale (Olaceae** **family)**

Jasmine is probably the most expensive oil of all, making it a real luxury. It is extracted from the delicate flowers which are picked by hand at night when their fragrance is at its most potent. The extraction process is necessarily complicated so that the flowers are not damaged; enfleurage was used originally, but jasmine oil available today is obtained by solvent extraction. The absolute is used extensively in perfumery, and indeed Ryman (1991, p. 116) suggests that today's jasmine oil is not suitable for therapeutic work partly because residual solvents will be found in the end-product. However, newer extraction methods such as the use of liquid carbon dioxide seem to have resolved the problem and most authorities continue to utilize jasmine, finding it useful in small doses of up to 2–3 per cent (International School of Aromatherapy, 1993, p. 98).

Worldwide production and availability currently exceed demand, so prices have fallen slightly in the early 1990s (Aqua Oleum, 1993). Jasmine absolute is available from Egypt, India, China, Morocco, France and Algeria, with Egypt producing the most and France and Algeria the least. Concerned practitioners may, however, wish to decline from purchasing Egyptian jasmine, for, although it is likely to be the least expensive, the lower costs are achieved at the expense of local children who are paid a pittance, insufficient even to feed them for a day, to collect the flowers (Aqua Oleum, 1993).

Chemical constituents There are well over 100 constituents in jasmine oil, which makes it difficult to synthesize, although its high price does lead to potential adulteration. It is, therefore, important to purchase the oil from a reputable supplier who can vouch for the authenticity of the batch from which you are buying.

There is a high level of the ketone jasmone found in the oil, which, together with methyl anthranilate, an ester, is responsible for the sweet heady aroma. Ketones are thought to be abortifacient so jasmine *should not be used in pregnancy* until term, in the absence of evidence to the contrary.

Esters of benzyl acetate, linalyl acetate and methyl anthranilate, and the ketones, are, however, antispasmodic so jasmine can be very useful in labour, during menstruation and, following delivery, for 'after pains'. It has a long tradition of use in childbirth by strengthening contractions and relieving pain (the ketones and the phenol, eugenol, are analgesic), as well as being a sedative yet mood-uplifting oil.

It is thought to be a hormone balancer and is particularly useful for mothers with depression who could drink jasmine tea or who could be given a massage with a blend containing jasmine oil. Work by Shrivastav *et al.* in 1988 and by Abraham *et al.* in 1979 demonstrated the potential value of jasmine flowers in suppressing lactation. As a hormone balancer for men it may be valuable in cases of infertility, by increasing production of spermatozoa, and it is well known for its aphrodisiac qualities, in cases of frigidity, impotence and premature ejaculation (Sellar, 1992, p. 81).

The oil's relaxing effect on the mind may be sedative (Davis, 1988; Lawless, 1992; Sellar, 1992), although Tisserand (1992) states that while it is a nerve sedative it is also uplifting, and Ryman (1991) acknowledges it as a stimulant. Certainly, research by Kikuchi *et al.* in 1989 demonstrated shortened sleeping times in mice and attributed the stimulant effects to *cis-* and *trans-*phytol.

The presence of alcohols in the form of benzyl, linalol, indol, farnesol, geraniol, nerol and terpineol give jasmine its considerable anti-infective properties, including antibacterial, antifungal and antiviral effects. It is thought to be useful for respiratory tract infections, due to the presence of the ketone, jasmone.

Dangers Jasmine has emmenagogic properties so *should not be used in pregnancy* until term. Its aroma can be overpowering for some people and overuse may result in a degree of narcosis: be guided by the personal preference of the mother. It is probably best not used in a vaporizer, except in extremely low dilutions intermittently, and because of the conflicting information regarding its sedative or stimulating effects it should be avoided at night. The cost may seem almost prohibitive to some midwives, even though the specific benefits in the care of newly delivered mothers outweigh this factor, but care must be taken that the product purchased is as pure as possible.

Blends Jasmine is a base note with a powerful aroma, but used in low doses will blend well with bergamot, cedarwood, camomile, clary sage, frankincense, geranium, grapefruit, lavender, lemongrass, mandarin, melissa, neroli, orange, rose, rosewood, sandalwood, tangerine and ylang ylang.

Juniper berry—
Juniperus
communis
(Cupressaceae
family)

Juniper berry essential oil, produced from *Juniperus communis*, must not be confused with other species of juniper, such as *J. virginiana* from which Virginian cedarwood oil is obtained, or *J. sabina* which produces savin oil. Both of these contain a different balance of chemicals which may be detrimental to a client for whom *J. communis* is appropriate.

The essential oil is extracted from the berries and other parts of the bush by steam distillation, producing a refreshing aroma with a hint of woodiness. Another oil is also produced from *J. communis*: juniper needle oil, which has a high sabinene content, whereas juniper berry is rich in α-pinene.

Chemical constituents The essential oil is rich in monoterpenes (camphene, pinene, myrcene, phellandrene and limonene) and in sesquiterpenes (cadinene, sabinene, cymene and terpinene). Together these chemicals result in juniper berry being useful as a disinfectant and antiseptic. The sesquiterpenes give it anti-inflammatory and antispasmodic properties, and help in lowering the blood pressure.

The main functions of juniper berry seem to be diuretic, probably due to an increase in the glomerular filtration rate, enabling more sodium and potassium to be excreted (Tisserand, 1992, p. 242). This means that it could be very useful in cases of severe ankle oedema in the postnatal period when the autolytic processes of involution, working faster than renal excretion, result in exacerbation of any pre-existing oedema. However, juniper berry is also an emmenagogue and should therefore *not* be be used for oedematous ankles during pregnancy, except *perhaps* near term (see below).

Juniper berry also contains alcohols such as borneol and terpineol, which add to the antibacterial and antiviral properties, as well as acting on the hepatic system which may help with detoxification of the liver, and it has apparently been used in cases of cirrhosis. Urinary tract infection in the puerperium may respond well to juniper berry in combination with other oils.

Dangers Juniper berry is known to be an emmenagogue and should be *avoided in pregnancy*, although Tisserand and Balacs (1995, p. 110) argue that this is not a reason for not using it. They cite several studies which refer to juniper generically and do not identify *J. communis* specifically. They acknowledge that juniper berries are known to be abortifacient but this does not seem to apply to the essential oil. A comprehensive discussion of their reasons for disputing the contraindication of juniper berries in pregnancy is given in their *Essential Oil Safety Guide* (1995, p. 142), but it is the belief of this author that, until more definite evidence is available, midwives should be extremely circumspect about the use of juniper berries during pregnancy, and ensure that they are using only *J. communis*.

The effects on the renal tract have not been fully investigated, and juniper berry should not be used on women who have a history of renal disease (International School of Aromatherapy, 1993, p. 65), including gestational hypertension. Overuse in women with no history of kidney disease may precipitate renal complications, although, again, Tisserand and Balacs (1995, p. 142) found no evidence against using it for people with kidney disease.

Prolonged use may result in allergy to the skin and respiratory tract, although the case reported by Rothe *et al.* in 1973 occurred after 25 years of occupational contact with products containing *J. communis*. Neat application of juniper berry oil may have approximately 2 per cent incidence of irritation (International School of Aromatherapy, 1993, p. 65).

Blends Juniper berry will blend well with benzoin, bergamot, cedarwood, clary sage, cypress, eucalyptus, frankincense, geranium, grapefruit, lemon, lime, melissa, orange, rosemary, sandalwood and thyme.

Lavender—
Lavandula
angustifolia
(Labiatae family)
Lavender is probably the most versatile essential oil used in aromatherapy and is produced by steam distillation from the flowers, and occasionally the stalks. The word 'lavender' originates from the Latin 'to wash', and the plant has a long worldwide tradition of medicinal usage as a cleanser. The quality of lavender varies according to the place in which it is grown, with some of the best coming from Grasse in France, the Alps, Norfolk in England and the former Yugoslavia.

There are, however, several types of lavender oil available and this is particularly important in midwifery. *Lavandula angustifolia*, sometimes known as *L. officinalis*, is the most odorous and the most commonly used therapeutic oil.

Midwives should always ask for the oil by its Latin name to avoid being offered one of the other types of lavender such as *L. stoechas*, *L. vera*, *L. dentata* (this latter is rich in 1.8 cineole as shown by Gamez *et al.*'s work in 1990) or even *L. spica* or *latifolia*, more usually called spike lavender. *L. intermedia, hortensis* and *burnatii* are terms that refer to essential oil of lavandin, obtained from a hybrid cross between *L. angustifolia* and *L. latifolia*. Lavandin oil is much cheaper to produce than lavender and is sometimes substituted for the latter, but the chemical constituents differ considerably. Other oils are occasionally mistaken for lavender: the cotton lavender is actually *Santolina chamaecyparissus*, belonging to an entirely different botanical family and having no use in aromatherapy because of its potential toxicity.

A trial by Buckle (1993) investigated the different effects of *L. officinalis* and *L. burnatii* on patients after cardiac surgery. She found that respiratory effects were similar but that *L. burnatii* appeared to be more effective in alleviating anxiety. It was noted that lavandin oil is rarely used (although trials into the antimyobacterial activity of lavandin have also been carried out by Gabbrielli *et al.* (1988)). While there were some flaws in the methodology of Buckle's trial, it was one of the first randomized double-blind controlled investigations in therapeutic aromatherapy and serves to demonstrate the importance of selecting essential oils by their Latin name rather than their common name.

Chemical constituents *L. angustifolia* contains alcohols such as linalol, borneol, geraniol and lavandulol, which together with some phenols makes it a strong anti-infective agent. Lavender is thought to be antibacterial, antifungal, antiviral and antimicrobial, and could be effective in reducing wound infection in mothers following Caesarean section or episiotomy. Dale and Cornwell's (1994) trial involving 635 women did not in fact demonstrate significant anti-infective effects of lavender oil used postepisiotomy, nor did there appear to be more rapid wound healing, another property attributed to lavender oil. However, the mothers did report a decrease in discomfort, and lavender is noted to be an effective analgesic, notably for headaches, due to its phenol and terpene (limonene, pinene and caryophyllene, a sesquiterpene) content. Consequently it can be useful in labour for easing contraction pain, and also acts as an antispasmodic due to the presence of esters such as geranyl acetate, lavandulyl acetate and linalyl acetate. Experience has shown that lavender oil massaged into the abdomen and back during labour seems to enhance and coordinate uterine action and can be effective where the placenta is slow to separate in the third stage of labour. In addition the phenols and esters produce a feeling of relaxation and sedation, as shown in Buchbauer *et al.'s* (1991) work.

Lavender oil is hypotensive due to the alcohols and sesquiterpenes, and can be valuable in late pregnancy and in labour where a mother has raised blood pressure. However, it should not be used for women with epidural anaesthesia *in situ* as it may compound the possible hypotensive effects of the bupivacaine.

Lavender oil contains a small amount of the ketone camphor, which can be emmenagogic, as well as some 1.8 cineole, an oxide, so, contrary to popular belief, lavender is *contraindicated in early pregnancy*, although some texts suggest that it may be used in small doses for conditions such as leucorrhoea. However, caution should be exercised in pregnancy, for percutaneous absorption of the oil into the blood has been demonstrated within 10 minutes of administration (Jager *et al.*, 1992). The expectorant action of the oxide content does, however, make lavender a good addition to an inhalation for respiratory tract congestion and infection.

Dangers As noted above lavender oil is *contraindicated in pregnancy* until almost term. Care should be taken that the oil used is *L. angustifolia*—be guided by price. Some dermal irritation has been reported (Brandao, 1986), although dermal toxicity of spike lavender (*L. spica*) is more than twice that of *L. angustifolia* (International School of Aromatherapy, 1993, p. 74), again emphasizing the need to be sure of the product being purchased.

The hypotensive action should be carefully monitored, and this, coupled with the sedating effects, may make some people feel drowsy after use. Certainly the hypotensive action precludes the use of lavender in women prone to postural hypotension or in those receiving epidural anaesthesia.

Blends Lavender has a very distinctive aroma, liked by most people, but some may prefer it to be subdued by blending with other oils. Lavender mixes well with basil, benzoin, bergamot, cedarwood, camomile, cinnamon, clary sage, cypress, eucalyptus, frankincense, geranium, grapefruit, jasmine, lemon, lemongrass, lime, mandarin, marjoram, melissa, neroli, nutmeg, orange, patchouli, petitgrain, rose, rosemary, rosewood, sandalwood, tangerine, thyme, tea tree and ylang ylang.

Lemon— *Citrus limon* Burman (Rutaceae family)

As might be expected, lemon essential oil has a lovely fresh citrussy aroma and is obtained by expression from the rind of the fruit. Ryman (1991, p. 129) states that production of lemon essence is second only to orange and that in 1987 2000–2500 tonnes of the oil were produced worldwide. This was superseded in 1991 when over 10,000 tonnes were produced (Aqua Oleum, 1993). Much of the therapeutic value of the oil can be obtained by ingesting the fruit or in part from drinking the juice, especially for its vitamin C content, but the essential oil has been used for many centuries as an antiseptic.

Chemical constituents　The principal constituent of lemon oil is limonene, a monoterpene, in quantities up to 70 per cent (Lawless, 1992, p. 119), or even 90 per cent (Ryman, 1991, p. 129), together with other monoterpenes myrcene, phellandrene and pinene, and some sesquiterpenes in the form of sabinene, cadinene, terpinene and β-bisabolene. The terpenes, in combination with alcohols (geraniol, linalol, octanol, nonalol) and the aldehyde, citral, mean that lemon is an extremely strong anti-infective oil, being antiseptic, antifungal, antibacterial and antiviral. The antifungal activity of the oil was investigated by Misra *et al.* in 1988, with citral being found to be the most effective component. It is also considered to be an immunostimulant, increasing the production of leucocytes, and may possibly improve erythrocyte vitality, thereby preventing anaemia.

The alcohols have a vasoconstrictive action and lemon has been used as a haemostatic agent in cases of haemorrhage. However, it is also thought to be a tonic to the circulatory system and may be effective in reducing hypertension, probably due to the alcohols, in conjunction with the coumarins and aldehydes. In addition, the coumarins seem to have an anticoagulant action, while the alcohols may act on the hepatic system.

Lemon does appear to work in almost a homoeopathic manner, for despite its acidic nature it can be helpful in reducing hyperacidity of the gastrointestinal tract. It is certainly known to be an effective laxative oil.

The fresh aroma is virtually universally pleasing and may act directly on the brain through the olfactory tract as an antidepressant and an uplift to the emotions, as demonstrated by Knasko's (1992) work.

Dangers Much has been written about the possible phototoxic effects of lemon essence, as well as other citrus essences, thought in this case to be due to the presence of bergapten and oxypeuce-danin (Naganuma *et al.*, 1985). Certainly lemon oil should not be used neat on the skin; dermatitis is possible in sensitive people, and low doses of about 1–2 per cent are recommended.

Oxidization can occur in lemon oil left exposed to oxygen or light, so it is best to buy small quantities of a good quality oil, ensuring that its shelf-life is still valid at the time of purchase.

Blends The fresh aroma of lemon essence will counteract some of the very heavy base aromas, and will blend well with benzoin, bergamot, black pepper, cedarwood, camomile, cypress, eucalyptus, frankincense, geranium, ginger, grapefruit, jasmine, juniper berry, lavender, mandarin, neroli, nutmeg, orange, patchouli, petitgrain, rose, sandalwood, tangerine, thyme, tea tree and ylang ylang.

Lemongrass— *Cymbopogon citratus* (Gramineae family) The oil is steam distilled from the grass, which is grown in the tropics, and much of the production is used by the food and perfumery industries. It is occasionally called Indian melissa or Indian verbena, but this must not be confused with *Melissa officinalis* or *Lippia citriodora* respectively.

Chemical constituents Lemongrass oil contains up to 85 per cent of the aldehyde citral, which is responsible for a strong antifungal and bactericidal action (Agarwal *et al.*, 1980; Onawunmi *et al.*, 1984; Onawunmi and Ogunlana, 1986; Ogunlana *et al.*, 1987; Onawunmi, 1988, 1989), although this is reduced by oxidization of the oil as a result of exposure to light, heat and oxygen (Orafidiya, 1993). Analgesia due to the monoterpenes, limonene and myrcene, has been demonstrated by Lorenzetti *et al.* (1991), while Seth *et al.* (1976) found the oil not only to relieve pain but also to be antipyretic and a central nervous system depressant. It is quoted as helping to eliminate lactic acid following exercise (Sellar, 1992, p. 92) and could be of use during labour and the postnatal period. It is also galactogogic, so may help in establishing lactation, although

Tisserand and Balacs (1995, p. 230) advise caution if the oil is administered orally to breastfeeding women.

Citral and the alcohol geraniol have been found to reduce serum cholesterol levels (Elson *et al.*, 1989) and lemongrass seems to have a carminative action, aiding digestion, stimulating appetite, relieving heartburn and easing flatulence. Other alcohols present include citronellol, farnesol, furfurol, geraniol, isopulegol, linalol, nerol and terpineol. Some anticarcinogenic qualities have been attributed to lemongrass oil, possibly because of the geraniol and *d*-limonene content (Zheng *et al.*, 1993).

Emotionally, the clean refreshing aroma of the oil seems to act in lifting the spirits and reviving energy. Lemongrass is an effective deodorant and insect repellant, and could be vaporized intermittently into the maternity department as an air freshener.

Dangers   Oxidization can occur fairly rapidly because of the high proportion of citral which changes to an acid and therefore affects the chemical profile of the oil, rendering it unsuitable for therapeutic work. There is some risk of dermal irritation as a result of the citral content so the oil should be used only in low dilutions.

Blends   Lemongrass blends well with basil, cedarwood, eucalyptus, geranium, jasmine, juniper berry, lavender, neroli, patchouli, rosemary and tea tree.

Lime—
Citrus aurantifolia
(Rutaceae family)   Lime is a much under-rated essential oil, and is valuable in midwifery as a member of the citrus group, with its fresh, sweet aroma, similar to bergamot. It should not be confused with lime blossom, sometimes called linden blossom (*Tilia europaea* or *cordata*), which is completely different. Unlike most citrus fruits, expression is not the principal method of extraction, although it may be used to produce oil for the perfumery industry; the essential oil for aromatherapy is normally obtained from the whole fruit by steam distillation, as the expressed product is phototoxic.

Chemical constituents   As might be expected, lime, in common with other citrus oils, contains limonene and other monoterpenes such as camphene and pinene as well as sequiterpenes in the form of sabinene and terpinoline. These give the oil strong antiseptic and anti-infective properties, and are also responsible for the

Plate 1 *Salvia sclarea* (clary sage).

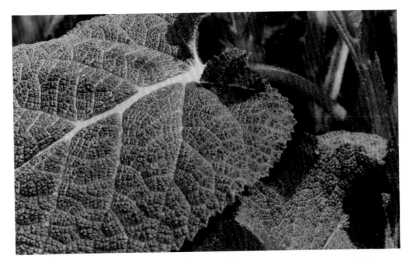

Plate 2 *Salvia officinalis* (sage). Note the difference between common garden sage and clary sage.

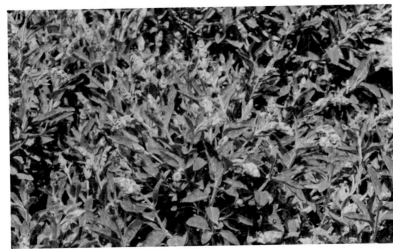

Plate 3 *Piper nigrum* (black pepper).

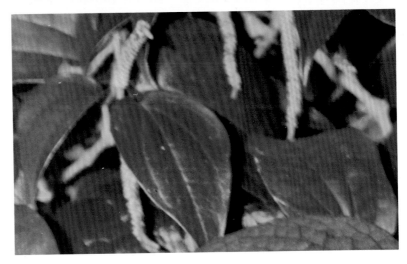

Plate 4 *Pelargonium officinalis* Graveolens (geranium).

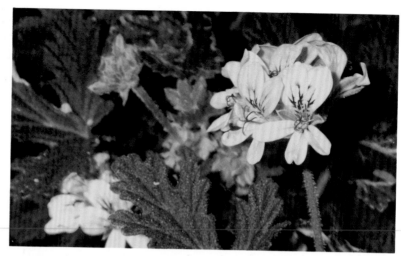

Plate 5 *Origanum vulgare* (marjoram).

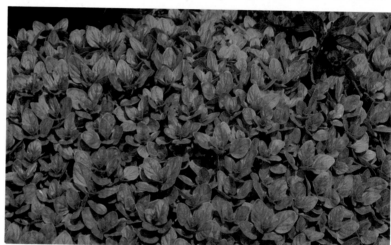

Plate 6 *Rosmarinus officinalis* (rosemary).

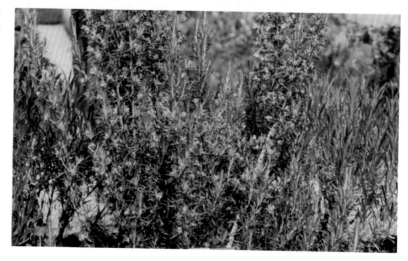

Plate 7 Woman receiving reflex zone therapy for stiff neck following epidural anaesthesia.

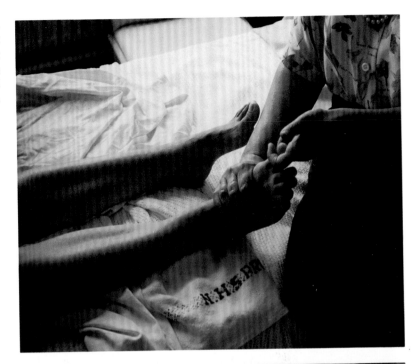

Plate 8 Woman receiving hand massage to reduce oedematous fingers.

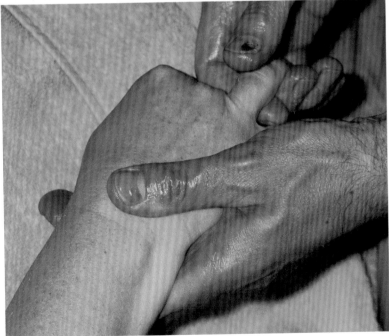

relaxing yet uplifting quality so easily evoked by simply inhaling the aroma.

The alcohols linalol and terpineol and the aldehyde citral also assist in the antibacterial, antiviral, antifungal and antiseptic actions of lime oil. In addition alcohols are thought to balance the immune system and act on the liver, possibly being useful in treating alcoholism (Sellar, 1992, p. 95). The terpenes, alcohols and aldehydes all contribute towards the relaxing effect of lime, while aldehydes and alcohols can help in reducing pyrexia.

Esters such as linalyl acetate, together with the sesquiterpenes, make lime oil anti-inflammatory and antispasmodic, so it is a good all-round choice for labour.

Lime is also used as an appetite regulator and could be beneficial for women with loss of appetite or with pica, as well as those suffering ptyalism.

Lime oil is considered safe to use throughout pregnancy (International School of Aromatherapy, 1993, p. 146) and could be blended with other citrus essences or alternated with them according to the woman's preference.

Dangers As with all citrus oils there is a risk of photosensitivity, although judicious use should reduce the potential dangers. High doses may irritate the skin in susceptible women.

Blends Lime oil blends well with all the other citrus essences such as bergamot, lemon, orange, mandarin, tangerine and petitgrain. It also complements citronella, clary sage, lavender, lemongrass, neroli, nutmeg, rose, rosemary and ylang ylang.

Mandarin—
Citrus nobilis
(Rutaceae family)

Mandarin has a lovely fresh citrus aroma reminiscent of the actual fruit and is obtained by cold expression from the outer peel. Mandarin is one of the most versatile and gentlest of essential oils and, as far as is known, is suitable for use on almost anyone receiving aromatherapy but particularly expectant mothers and children.

Chemical constituents Mandarin essence has a bluish tinge due to the presence of methylanthranilate, an ester which makes it a good antiseptic. It has an affinity with the gastrointestinal tract, being carminative, digestive and laxative as a result of the esters. The aldehydes citral and citronellal and the alcohol geraniol provide the anti-infective properties of the essence. In addition geraniol assists diuresis while the esters are antispasmodic. A small amount of the monoterpene limonene gives mandarin essence analgesic properties but is also responsible for the potential to cause skin irritation. Conversely it can be useful in reducing the tendency to striae gravidarum and scarring. Like all citrus essences, mandarin is thought to be slightly phototoxic but this has not been shown to be significant.

Mandarin's refreshing aroma is almost universally acceptable and, as it is safe and versatile, it can be used on virtually all clients except those allergic to citrus friut. The terpenes act as a stimulant and mild antidepressant, the latter characteristic being enhanced by the phenols.

Dangers   As mentioned above, mandarin may be phototoxic if used undiluted and could cause some skin irritation in sensitive people, but is otherwise one of the safest essences to use in aromatherapy. Care should, however, be taken, as with all essential oils, not to use it continuously throughout pregnancy; in labour its use should be intermittent and midwives should consider discontinuing it if the mother is having an emotionally unsatisfying labour, in an attempt to prevent long-term olfactory association of mandarin with an unpleasant situation.

Blends   Mandarin blends well with many essential oils including basil, bergamot, black pepper, camomile, grapefruit, lavender, lemon, lemongrass, lime, marjoram, neroli, nutmeg, petitgrain, rose, rosemary, sandalwood, tea tree and ylang ylang.

Marjoram—
Origanum
marjorana
(Labiatae family)

This oil, with its warm, spicy and somewhat medicinal aroma, is produced by distillation from the flowers and leaves of the plant (Plate 5). It has a long tradition of use as a medicine, especially for stomach upsets.

Chemical constituents   The alcohols, borneol, linalol, pinocarvol and α-terpineol, mean that marjoram is a good anti-infective agent, being antibacterial, antifungal and antiviral, as well as an immune system balancer. They also act directly on the hepatic system, helping to stimulate and aid liver and biliary function, and can be helpful in alleviating constipation and abdominal colic. The monoterpene pinene and the sesquiterpenes sabinene and β-caryophyllene assist in relieving pain, especially muscular discomfort following exercise, and headache. Camphor, a ketone, is a valuable expectorant, so is useful for colds, influenza and bronchitis, but is also an emmenagogue so marjoram *should be avoided in pregnancy*, except in very small doses towards term.

Aldehydes, in the form of citral and geranyl acetate, add to the anti-infective qualities of the oil, and also lower the blood pressure; this is enhanced by the large number of alcohols. In addition, aldehydes help to lower temperature, and are relaxing, but may be responsible for skin irritation.

Phenolic glycosides, arbutin and hydroquinone, have been found in Egyptian marjoram oil, and the latter component showed some cytotoxic activity against cultured rat cells (Assaf *et al.*, 1987).

Dangers Marjoram should be *avoided in pregnancy* as insufficient information is known about its emmenagogic properties. The relaxing effects may be sufficient to cause drowsiness, so care should be taken when using marjoram that the client is not about to drive a vehicle.

When purchasing the oil it is important not to confuse *Origanum marjorana* (commonly called sweet marjoram) with Spanish marjoram (*Thymus mastichina*), which has a much higher 1.8 cineole content, sometimes up to 75 per cent.

Blends Marjoram has a warm camphorous aroma which blends well with basil, bergamot, cedarwood, camomile, clary sage, cypress, lavender, lemon, mandarin, melissa, nutmeg, orange, peppermint, rosewood and sandalwood.

Neroli—
Citrus aurantium
or *bigaradia*
(Rutaceae family)

This is one of the most expensive and luxurious essential oils, derived from the delicate petals of the bitter orange tree by a process of solvent extraction or occasionally steam distillation from the freshly picked flowers—a tonne of flowers is needed to produce just one kilogram of oil, hence the price.

Chemical constituents Neroli contains a high proportion of alcohols (linalol, nerol, nerolidol, farnesol, indol, terpineol and geraniol), as well as esters such as linalyl acetate, methyl anthranilate, geranyl acetate, benzyl acetate and neryl acetate. There is a small amount of the ketone, jasmone and some monoterpenes in the form of limonene, α- and β-pinene, and camphene.

The main value of neroli appears to be reduction of stress, a result of the relaxing properties of the esters, aldehydes and ketones, and the hypotensor effects of the alcohols and aldehydes. Stevenson's (1992) controlled trial with patients in intensive care demonstrated that relaxation and reduction in anxiety could be obtained from a 10-minute foot massage using neroli.

Jager *et al.* (1992) also demonstrated reduced motility, i.e. sedation, in mice. This oil could certainly be used in late pregnancy in small doses, and particularly in labour to alleviate tension and stress. Ryman (1991, p. 155) recommends its use for premenstrual tension, and this could equally apply to postnatal 'blues' and depression. The esters are responsible for neroli being antispasmodic, which may be further justification for its use during labour, involution and subsequent menstruation.

Neroli has been quoted as being aphrodisiac (Lawless, 1992, p. 144), possibly as a result of the relaxation obtained, and this would make it a suitable oil for women to use after the puerperium when their libido may not have returned to normal.

For insomnia during late pregnancy or the puerperium neroli is a special oil to add to a blend, although it can have a rather hypnotic effect on some people.

The toning effect on the circulatory system is possibly due to the high level of alcohols, and neroli seems to assist in promoting healthy skin. During late pregnancy abdominal massage with neroli oil *may* prevent striae gravidarum, and can promote wound healing and cell regeneration in the postnatal period.

Dangers Neroli is thought to be safe to use in pregnancy but it is advisable to blend it in low dilutions owing to the presence of a small amount of jasmone, and to administer it only towards term. The relaxation achieved can be soporific and hypnotic, so women should not drive immediately after receiving it.

Blends Neroli is a base note with an aroma that takes a while to warm up and which lingers longer than many other orangey aromas. It blends well with basil, bergamot, cedarwood, camomile, citronella, geranium, jasmine, lemon, lemongrass, lime, mandarin, melissa, orange, patchouli, petitgrain, rose, sandalwood, tangerine and ylang ylang.

Nutmeg—
Myristica fragrans
(Myristicaceae
family)

Essential oil of nutmeg is obtained from the seed kernels by steam distillation and has a warm spicy, rather sharp, aroma. Britain is quoted (Ryman, 1991, p. 158) as being the second largest consumer of nutmeg oil in the world. The essential oil should be very pale yellow with a thin consistency; if it has turned dark brown, thick and has a more unpleasant aroma, it should not be used for therapeutic work.

Chemical constituents   Nutmeg oil contains between 1 and 14 per cent of the phenol myristicine, depending on its source. This can not only cause severe skin irritation but is also narcotic, hallucinogenic and toxic, and for this reason the oil should certainly *never be used in pregnancy*—the fact that it is also an emmenagogue is less significant than the overall toxicity of the oil. Tisserand and Balacs (1995, p. 107) dispute this and suggest that administration via massage is acceptable, there being insufficient proof regarding the need to avoid it during pregnancy. It is, however, this very lack of evidence that should govern its use—or lack of use—in midwifery practice.

Other phenols present include safrole, which is potentially carcinogenic, and eugenol, so that nutmeg is a powerful anti-infective oil. Bennett *et al.*'s work (1988) demonstrated that the eugenol reduces muscle tone in the gastrointestinal tract and myometrium, and inhibits prostaglandin synthesis. It also appears to have anti-inflammatory effects and has been used for many years as an effective treatment for diarrhoea. Later investigations by Janssens *et al.* (1990) showed that eugenol and isoeugenol are effective in inhibiting platelet aggregation, but they recommended that, to prevent the side-effects of nutmeg oil, synthetic preparations of the active ingredients should be used in preference.

The carminative, laxative phenols generally mean that nutmeg is good for digestive complaints, including both diarrhoea and constipation.

Various alcohols (about 4–8 per cent according to Lawless (1992, p. 139)) such as geraniol, borneol, linalol, cymol, sapol, globulol and terpineol add to the antibacterial, antiviral and antifungal properties, and act as an immune system balancer. Alcohols are also vasoconstrictive and nutmeg is known to be a cardiac stimulant, so should never be used in high doses.

Up to 88 per cent of the oil is comprised of the monoterpenes camphene, dipentene, pinene, limonene and phellandrene, and the sesquiterpenes, α-terpenene and sabinene, which give nutmeg strong analgesic properties that seem especially effective for uterine pain in labour or for dysmenorrhoea; indeed, nutmeg has a tradition in some cultures of being used for childbearing women. However, Tisserand and Balacs (1995, p. 153) cite research which demonstrates that nutmeg's main constituent, myristicin, inhibits monoamine oxidase, although this is less significant in the whole essential oil. However, monoamine oxidase inhibitors should not be given in conjunction with pethidine (Reynolds, 1993; cited by Tisserand and Balacs, 1995, p. 153), so if nutmeg oil is used during labour the midwife should make the mother aware that she will not be able to resort to pethidine at a later stage. It is also good for other muscular aches and pains, notably rheumatic and dental pain. The presence of the oxide 1.8 cineole means that the oil is expectorant and mucolytic.

As an anti-stress remedy nutmeg has been used for many years, and recently an American company has patented the oil following investigations into its use in reducing blood pressure (Aqua Oleum, 1993).

Dangers The myristicin content of nutmeg oil makes it potentially lethal in aromatherapy. It is included here because, in experienced hands, small doses of the oil can be of use during labour, except in women also receiving pethidine. Many texts on aromatherapy seem to contradict one another as to the safety of nutmeg oil, but with the current level of knowledge it is advised that it should *not be used in pregnancy* and the maximum dilution recommended is 2 per cent in fit healthy adults.

Tests on animals have shown central nervous system paralysis and fatty degeneration of the liver (Balacs, 1993); intoxication in humans can lead to nausea and vomiting, tachycardia, visual impairment, stupor, epileptiform fits and hallucinations (International School of Aromatherapy, 1993, p. 79). Farrell (1994a) cites the report of a 25-year-old man with acute psychosis as a result of chronic nutmeg abuse. The danger of ingesting the oil should be remembered, too, when storing it, particularly when in the home, for overdose in a child could be fatal. It is interesting to note that mice given large amounts of Coca-Cola, which also contains myristicin, developed hepatic problems associated with carcinogenicity, although the researchers did point out that there is no direct evidence of the carcinogenic tendency of myristicin-containing essential oils (Balacs, 1993).

Blends Nutmeg can be used in small doses by experienced aromatherapists and blends well with black pepper, cinnamon, clary sage, cypress, frankincense, geranium, lemon, lime, mandarin, melissa, orange, patchouli, petitgrain, rosemary and tea tree.

**Orange, sweet—
Citrus sinensis
(Rutaceae family)**

Sweet orange is one of the safest and most versatile of all the essences and can be used during pregnancy and for children. It is obtained from the rind by cold expression or steam distillation, but, because it can oxidize quickly, antioxidants are usually added.

A similar oil is obtained from the bitter orange peel (*Citrus aurantium*) but the larger amount of coumarins increases the potential phototoxic effects of the bitter orange essence.

Chemical constituents As with other citrus essences, sweet orange contains over 90 per cent of monoterpenes, mainly limonene, with some camphene, myrcene and the sesquiterpene sabinene. These assist in the antiseptic and antibacterial qualities of sweet orange but also contribute towards the possible skin irritation that may occur in some people when sweet orange is used in high doses.

Aldehydes in the form of citral, together with the esters methyl anthranilate and neryl acetate, some coumarins and alcohols (fenchol, terpineol, linalol and nerol) make orange a relaxing essence and a mood uplifter, suitable for administration to women with hypertension, insomnia, anxiety, stress and depression. It is possible that it could be of value for hypercholesterolaemia.

Sweet orange is one of the most valuable essences to use for digestive complaints including nausea and vomiting, especially of biliary aetiology, constipation, diarrhoea, lack of appetite and possibly weight loss through its effect on fats. It can be used for babies with colic too.

The vitamin C content is obviously helpful for colds and influenza, although it would be better to eat whole oranges or drink the fresh juice. However, the essence may be effective in reducing pyrexia, probably by inducing sweating.

The essence can have a beneficial action on the skin and may help to prevent or reduce the severity of striae gravidarum, dry skin and dermatitis.

The analgesic effects of the monoterpenes indicate orange essence's value in labour. It is thought to reduce oedema, so could be good to use in late pregnancy and in the early puerperium for swollen ankles and feet (it is certainly safer than some other oils used to reduce oedema), and could be used during the premenstrual phase or the menopause.

Dangers   Sweet orange is extremely versatile and, as far as is known, safe to use in almost anyone. However, it should not be used in people who are allergic to citrus fruit. Neither should its versatility lead to prolonged use, as no oil should be used continuously for more than 3 weeks.

Care should be taken to purchase *Citrus sinensis* and to ensure it is as organic as possible, for many crops of oranges are sprayed with chemicals to improve their colour, or with wax to help retain moisture. Only small quantities of the essence should be purchased as it will deteriorate quickly and must be stored in a cool dark place with the lid of the bottle firmly in place. When blending, only the amount required should be mixed and any left over discarded.

There is a risk of skin irritation in some women with sensitive skins, and phototoxicity may be a problem if the woman goes into bright sunlight immediately after administration, although it is likely that the effects last no longer than 2 hours.

Blends   The refreshing, sweet and familiar aroma of oranges is pleasing to almost everyone. However, care should be taken as to how it is used, especially during labour, for if labour and delivery are difficult or unsatisfying for the mother, she may reject oranges for life.

Sweet orange blends well with basil, benzoin, bergamot, camomile, cinnamon, clary sage, cypress, frankincense, geranium, ginger, grapefruit, jasmine, juniper berry, lavender, lemon, lemongrass, lime, mandarin, marjoram, neroli, nutmeg, patchouli, petitgrain, rose, rosemary, rosewood, sandalwood, tangerine, tea tree and ylang ylang.

Patchouli—
Pogostemon
patchouli
(Labiatae family)

Patchouli oil is extracted from the leaves by steam distillation, and the heavy sweet aroma improves with age, lingering for a long time once used (hence it is a base note, often used in perfumery as a fixative). It may be a yellowish brown in colour or a deep reddish brown due to iron deposits oxidized from the metal containers in which it is stored when distilled in its country of origin (Seychelles, Indonesia, China and India). Patchouli has a long tradition of use in Chinese and Indian medicine and some readers may recall the 'Swinging Sixties' when it was often burned as incense with sandalwood and jasmine.

Chemical constituents   About 40 per cent of the oil is comprised of the alcohol patchoulol, and there are around 18 per cent esters. Sesquiterpenes in the form of patchoulene, caryophyllene and cadinene, aldehydes such as benzoic and cinnamic aldehyde, and the phenol eugenol make up the bulk of the remaining constituents. There is also a small amount of the ketone carvone present in the oil and up to 40 per cent patchouli camphor in the dried leaves (Ryman, 1991, p. 171). Davis (1988, p. 259) notes that patchoulene has a similar chemical structure to azulene, produced from camomile during the extraction process, which may account for the comparable anti-inflammatory properties of patchouli.

The oil can be sedative in action when used in low doses but may have the reverse effect when the concentration is too high. Some authorities suggest it has aphrodisiac properties and can help in increasing libido, while others question this as the aroma can be unpleasant for some people, especially in larger doses. It is often quoted as being an antidepressant.

Patchouli oil appears to be effective for use on the skin, easing allergies and eczema, and helping with wound healing when the skin is cracked, possibly by encouraging tissue regeneration and scar formation. The anti-infective properties are particularly useful for fungal infections of the skin such as athlete's foot, and for scalp conditions such as dandruff. It may also be of help for haemorrhoids.

Several authorities believe patchouli oil can be effective in treating obesity by curbing appetite, acting as a diuretic and preventing fluid retention and cellulite. It has been used for both diarrhoea by toning the gastrointestinal tract and for constipation by stimulating a sluggish colon (Tisserand, 1992, p. 264).

Dangers   Ryman comments (1991, p. 171) that no research has been undertaken to evaluate the effects of the iron that leaches from the metal containers used for storage, or of the second distillation often carried out by perfumers in an attempt to alter the colour, on the therapeutic actions of the final oil. Occasionally the oil may be adulterated with others such as cedar or cubebs, or with synthetic caryophyllene.

Care should be taken with dosage to ensure the correct balance and to avoid stimulating the central nervous system when sedation is the required effect.

No authorities appear to have questioned the use of patchouli specifically during pregnancy and it is not considered to be an emmenagogue, but it would be wise to be cognisant of the various effects and to use the oil sparingly.

Blends   The aroma of patchouli may be too heavy for some women and the therapist should be guided by the preference of the individual. The oil blends well with bergamot, black pepper, clary sage, frankincense, geranium, ginger, lavender, lemongrass, neroli, orange, rose, rosewood and sandalwood.

Petitgrain—
Citrus bigaradia
(Rutaceae family)

Petitgrain essential oil is extracted by steam distillation from the leaves and twigs of the bitter orange tree from which neroli is also derived, and contemporary supplies come from Paraguay, although small quantities of a better quality oil still come from France. The essential oil is used extensively in both the perfumery and the food industries, but not a great deal in aromatherapy. However, it does have some therapeutic values and, as far as is known, is safe to use in pregnancy.

Chemical constituents   The oil contains up to 80 per cent esters such as linalyl acetate, geranyl acetate, neryl acetate and terpenyl acetate, but oxidization can cause these to convert to acids so care must be taken to store the oil appropriately. The esters act as a balancer and are useful for inducing a sense of relaxation and lifting the mood, making petitgrain a good oil for women with mood swings, stress and anxiety. It can help insomnia and restlessness, possibly by easing respiration and relaxing the muscles (Sellar, 1992, p. 129). It seems to have a soothing action on the emotions, especially in cases of panic, and could be useful for the transition stage of labour.

Several alcohols are found in the oil including linalol, nerol, geraniol, terpineol, farnesol, nerolidol and citronellol, and these together with the esters and the terpenes, limonene and camphene, give the oil antibacterial, antifungal, antiviral and general antiseptic properties. It has been used for acne and other skin disorders and may be a suitable oil for women who develop a greasy skin during pregnancy, administered as a facial sauna. It can also be added to the rinsing water for greasy hair and may help when a pregnant woman perspires excesively due to the physiological rise in temperature.

A small proportion of the aldehyde citral assists in the anti-infective qualities and, with the alcohols, acts as a hypotensive and temperature-reducing agent.

As with many other of the citrus essences, petitgrain can be effective in treating constipation, flatulence and indigestion, an action that is probably enhanced when blending a synergistic mix of petitgrain and orange, mandarin or neroli.

Dangers Petitgrain oil is thought to be non-toxic, non-irritant and non-sensitizing, although this latter is contentious as a small number of subjects with existing dermatological conditions have been found to become sensitive to it and it is recommended that very low dilutions are used for these clients (International School of Aromatherapy, 1993, p. 65).

Blends Petitgrain blends well with other citrus oils such as bergamot, sweet orange, neroli, grapefruit and mandarin, as well as with benzoin, citronella, clary sage, geranium, lavender, jasmine, rosemary, rosewood, sandalwood and ylang ylang.

Rose—
Rosa damascena,
***centifolia* and**
***gallica* (Rosaceae**
family)

Rose oil is amongst the most luxurious in the world and, together with jasmine and neroli, is one of the most expensive. Although there are several hundred species and hybrids of rose, only three main species are used for essential oil production as these are the most aromatic. *Rosa damascena*, grown in Bulgaria, is steam distilled then decanted to separate the oil from the water and so produce rose otto or attar; a rose absolute is produced through solvent extraction (previously through enfleurage) from *R. centifolia* in France; more commonly nowadays a hybrid of *R. centifolia* and *R. gallica*, called rose de mai, is grown to produce an absolute or concrete (Lawless, 1992, p. 157). Roses are extremely sensitive to climatic changes and some crops produce oils of superior quality while others are not so good. The absolutes are not generally used for therapeutic work as essential oils are steam distilled from the original extract and are more suited to aromatherapy.

When buying rose essential oil it is wise to be guided by price to a certain extent, for it takes the petals of approximately 60,000 roses to produce one ounce of the oil (Tisserand, 1992, p. 272).

Roses and their aroma are pleasing to almost everyone, and such is the plant's popularity that a Rose Museum has been established near Frankfurt, the only one of its kind in the world, devoted to collecting, exhibiting and researching this marvellous flower (Kubler and Wabner, 1994).

Chemical constituents   The chemical constituents of the different types of rose oil are similar, although the balance of these chemicals may vary significantly depending on soil, weather, geography and the method of extraction. There are over 300 constituents of rose which have been identified, even though some of them are in negligible amounts. However, Brud and Konopacka-Brud (1994) suggest that the aroma and the therapeutic properties may depend on the ratios of these minor constituents.

Citronellol (around 20 per cent) and phenyl ethanol (up to 60 per cent), eugenol, farnesol, geraniol, linalol and nerol, which are alcohols, are present in varying amounts and contribute towards the anti-infective and immunostimulant properties of rose oil. The vasoconstrictive and astringent actions of the alcohols help in controlling haemostasis, and rose oil can be effective for a variety of skin conditions.

The rose seems to have a great affinity with the female reproductive tract and, with its lovely feminine aroma, is particularly suited to use in midwifery and gynaecological care. Rose oil may be used to regulate the menstrual cycle, for premenstrual tension and the menopause, menorrhagia, dysmenorrhoea, leucorrhoea and post-hysterectomy syndrome. In labour it can be very relaxing and can aid uterine action. However, while Tisserand and Balacs (1995, p. 111) disagree that its emmenagogic actions preclude its use during pregnancy, it would be wise to be cautious and avoid administration until almost term. Postnatally it can be a lovely addition to a massage or a bath oil, perhaps combined with jasmine for a real luxury.

Digestive and hepatic conditions can be treated, such as biliary nausea, constipation and even cholecystitis, according to Lawless (1992, p. 159). Holmes (1994) attributes this to the cooling, drying nature of the oil, as defined in Chinese and traditional Greek medicine.

However, the main value of rose oil is in relieving stress-related conditions, including tension, insomnia and depression, possibly as a result of the balancing action of the oil's effect on the hypothalamus (Holmes (1994) quotes nearly 30 emotions that may respond to rose oil). The relaxing and aphrodisiac qualities can be helpful for frigidity and impotence caused by emotional factors, and may trigger the release of dopamine from the brain (Sellar, 1992, p. 135).

Dangers   It is vital, when purchasing rose oil, to ensure it is of the highest possible quality, although this can be confirmed only by chromatography. (Reputable suppliers may provide a printout of the analysis.) A variety of synthetic chemicals may be used to adulterate the oil, or additions of other oils that smell similar and contain similar chemical constituents, such as rose geranium, may be found in the retailed product.

When an absolute is produced, chemical solvents are used, traces of which may be found in the final extract. This is important as most of the readily available rose oil will be an absolute, for up to six times more absolute can be extracted than essential oil (Holmes, 1994).

Blends   Rose is classed as having a middle to base note, from a perfumery point of view, and tends to be a subtle addition to a blend, with the main strength of the aroma becoming evident after it has warmed. It blends well with benzoin, bergamot, camomile, cedarwood, clary sage, geranium, grapefruit, jasmine, lavender, lemon, lime, mandarin, melissa, neroli, sweet orange, patchouli, rosewood, tangerine, sandalwood and ylang ylang.

Rosemary— *Rosmarinus officinalis* (Labiatae family)   This oil has a strong herbal and quite penetrating camphorous aroma and has a long tradition of medicinal usage. It is steam distilled from the flowers and leaves, but a poorer quality oil is also obtained from the whole plant, primarily in Spain (Plate 6).

Chemical constituents   As might be expected from the aroma, rosemary contains a small amount of camphor, which is a ketone, and another of this group, thujone, making the oil potentially abortifacient and therefore *contraindicated in pregnancy*, although it could be used in small doses near term. Indeed, Tisserand and Balacs (1995, p. 111) suggest that rosemary is safe to use externally, in massage, but should not be administered internally during pregnancy. The ketones, together with almost 50 per cent of the oxide 1.8 cineole, account for the expectorant, decongestant and mucolytic properties, so that rosemary can be extremely effective in clearing the head in people with colds and influenza.

The cephalic effects (stimulating and energizing the mind) have long been known, and indeed Shakespeare's 'rosemary for remembrance' helps to remind us of one of the uses for this oil. Kovar *et al.* (1987) demonstrated the stimulating effects of oil of rosemary in mice, although they were not able to attribute this effect to any individual component. Midwives on night duty could consider putting two drops on a handkerchief to sniff in order to keep them alert and awake! Postnatally rosemary could be given to an exhausted mother as a temporary relief, especially if she has tension headaches or mild 'blues'.

Monoterpenes and sesquiterpenes in the form of camphene, limonene, pinene and β-caryophyllene contribute to the analgesic action, which is particularly effective for muscular aches and pains and could be useful for women in labour or for dysmenorrhoea. Premenstrually and postnatally it may help to reduce oedema.

Various alcohols (borneol, terpineol and linalol) assist in the generally anti-infective value of the essential oil, and the stimulating and uplifting actions. A partial antimicrobial action was demonstrated by Soliman *et al.* (1994), who found the oil effective against *Mycobacterium intracellulare*, *Candida albicans* and *Cryptococcus neoformans* but not against *Staphylococcus aureus*, *Escherichia coli*, *Pseudomonas aeruginosa* and others.

The alcohols are responsible for a vasoconstrictive effect and it is probably for this reason that rosemary is a hypertensive oil: it may be beneficial for women with hypotension but should be avoided in those with raised blood pressure. The astringency contributes to wound healing, and interestingly Tisserand (1992, p. 281) states that the Arabs apply the powdered herb, as an antiseptic and haemostatic, to the umbilical cords of newborn babies.

Rosemary is a component of many proprietary hair-care products and the oil can be added to rinsing water for greasy hair, and used in a variety of scalp and hair disorders such as dandruff, seborrhoea and thinning hair—helpful for women whose hair thins during pregnancy or, more often, in the months following delivery.

A small amount of the antispasmodic ester bornyl acetate helps gastrointestinal discomforts such as flatulence, colic (but best avoided in babies), dyspepsia and possibly gallbladder problems. This spasmolytic activity is thought to be a result of acetylcholine antagonism (Taddei *et al.*, 1988; Aqel 1991). Al-Hader *et al.* (1994) also found that rosemary oil increased blood glucose and decreased insulin levels in rabbits.

Dangers Rosemary essential oil is potentially abortifacient so *should be used sparingly during pregnancy.* It is contraindicated in women who are hypertensive, with either essential hypertension or pre-eclampsia; it should not be used by epileptics, although very small amounts may work homoeopathically to treat epilepsy (Davis, 1988, p. 293).

Adulteration with turpentine oils or another essential oil such as sage may occur, so careful purchasing is necessary to ensure purity. The strong aroma may antidote homoeopathic remedies.

Blends Rosemary's strong camphorous aroma blends well with basil, cedarwood, frankincense, geranium, ginger, grapefruit, lavender, lime, mandarin, melissa, orange, petitgrain, tangerine and thyme.

Rosewood—
Aniba rosaeodora
(Lauraceae family)

This essential oil, extracted by steam distillation from the wood chippings, has only recently come into use in aromatherapy, although its continued use is in doubt, for the trees originate in the Brazilian rain forests and are being extensively felled for wood. Midwives concerned about environmental issues should be aware that its production is reputed to be contributing to the damage resulting from deforestation, and they may therefore wish to refrain from its use. However, rosewood oil is also available from Peru and Guyana and, although the crop is smaller and there are logistical problems of transportation which increase the price, rosewood oil from these countries does not interfere with the environment. Additionally the harvesting is controlled and replanting is actively encouraged (Aqua Oleum, 1993).

Chemical constituents One of the main constituents is the alcohol, linalol (about 80–97 per cent according to its country of origin), with geraniol, nerol, terpineol. These, and the terpenes, limonene, pinene and terpinene, mean that the oil has anti-infective properties, immunostimulant action (due to the alcohols) and some mild analgesic effects (terpenes).

The alcohols and a small amount of the aldehyde citronellal make it relaxing, mood uplifting and hypotensive, although it may also have a stimulating action and is therefore considered to be a balancer. It is of value as an aphrodisiac, anti-stress remedy and for nervous tension symptoms such as headache and nausea. McCardle (1992) reported its benefits in reducing blood pressure in a woman with fulminating pre-eclampsia.

Skin conditions seem to respond fairly well to rosewood and it may have a part to play in wound healing, prevention of striae gravidarum and even ageing skin.

Dangers   Some aromatherapists believe that rosewood can be substituted with Ho wood oil as the linalol content is similar, but this is not appropriate for the balance of other constituents will be different; Price (1993, p. 114) suggests experimenting with Ho wood (*Cinnamomum camphora*) for its *similar aroma* or even with rhodium wood oil (*Convolvulus scoparius*, often referred to as 'rosewood', and usually found as a blend of geranium or palmarosa combined with sandalwood). While, in principle, Price may have a point in that these alternatives may achieve the desired therapeutic effects without using true rosewood oil, it seems somewhat irresponsible to advise these substitutions for clinical work. Furthermore it again emphasizes the need for aromatherapists to adopt the practice of referring to oils by their Latin names rather than their common names so that the correct, most appropriate, oil may be selected. It is not good practice either to use a synthetic form of linalol for therapeutic work, and midwives and aromatherapists should ensure that they purchase their *Aniba rosaeodora* from a reputable supplier and not from a perfume source.

Blends   Rosewood blends well with cajuput, cedarwood, frankincense, geranium, grapefruit, jasmine, mandarin, marjoram, orange, patchouli, petitgrain, rose, rosemary, sandalwood, tangerine and ylang ylang.

Sandalwood—
Santalum album
(Santalaceae
family)

Most commercially available sandalwood oil comes from trees grown in the Mysore region of India, all of which are now owned and controlled by the Indian government as a conservationary measure, although, until the replanting process results in more established trees, this has served only to increase the price artificially. Consequently many buyers of sandalwood oil have turned to Indonesia and China, and some oil comes from New Caledonia but is very expensive owing to transportation costs.

Another type of sandalwood (*Eurcarya spicata* or *Santalum spicatum*) is grown in Australia and, although this is a very effective agent against Gram-positive bacteria, *Staphylococcus aureus* and *Candida albicans*, it is currently a protected species and therefore the oil is not available commercially (International School of Aromatherapy,

1993, p. 63). Sandalwood oil is extracted by steam distillation from wood chips from the inner heartwood and the roots, and allowed to mature for up to 6 months, when it is re-distilled under vacuum to produce an oil suitable for use, the initial distillate being too crude.

Chemical constituents The main constituent is a mixture of two sesquiterpenic alcohols, called santalol (around 90 per cent). Other alcohols such as borneol and teresantol, approximately 6 per cent santalene and other sesquiterpenes, and the aldehyde furfurol are also present. Jirovetz *et al.*'s (1992) investigations in which blood samples from mice that had inhaled sandalwood oil were analysed, showed α-santalol, β-santalol and α-santalene to be present in significant amounts; when given pure fragrance compounds, the blood analyses also showed the presence of coumarins and α-terpineol.

The oil's principal value lies in its affinity with the genitourinary and respiratory systems, and with the gastrointestinal tract. Sandalwood is extremely effective in combating cystitis and urinary tract infections, as well as genital discharges, for example leucorrhoea and gonorrhoea. Massage of the oil into the suprapubic and sacral areas has an anti-inflammatory and anti-infective effect, and is generally soothing. In the case of gonorrhoea, Tisserand (1992, p. 284) surmises that sandalwood's action is not due directly to an antibacterial effect, but that it 'abolishes spontaneous contractions of the spermatic cord, lessens the motility of the genital tract muscles, has a diuretic effect and inhibits secretions'. However, as Davis (1988, p. 299) points out, while it may have been used for conditions such as cystitis and gonorrhoea for over 2500 years in traditional medicine, it would be illegal, i.e. contrary to the Cancer Act, for an aromatherapist to use it as the sole treatment without medical training, although it may be useful in conjunction with conventional care after consultation with medical staff.

Expectoration and reduction in sputum production can be achieved by administering sandalwood as an inhalation; it can be of benefit for bronchitis, coughs, colds, catarrh and sore throats, partly through the mucolytic and decongestant actions but also due to the antiseptic property. A facial sauna can effectively treat acne and greasy skin.

Sandalwood is a very relaxing oil, which may account for its well-known aphrodisiac quality; certainly the aroma is pleasing to both men and women, and it may be of assistance in treating puerperal frigidity or impotence when there is an underlying psychological cause. The astringency of sandalwood may help in combating diarrhoea, and it has been used to good effect for nausea and vomiting and for heartburn.

Dangers   The prohibitive cost and limited availability of pure, legal, sandalwood oil often leads to its adulteration with other oils such as palm, linseed or castor, or with essential oils, e.g. guaiacwood or cedarwood. Midwives who are concerned should enquire from their supplier as to the quality and source of the oil.

Sellar (1992, p. 143) suggests that the potency of the relaxation effect of the oil precludes its use in people who are pathologically depressed as it may lower their mood even further, making them completely introspective.

Blends   Sandalwood's aroma is a base note and it lingers for a considerable length of time after use. The oil blends well with basil, benzoin, black pepper, clary sage, cypress, frankincense, geranium, jasmine, juniper berry, lavender, lemon, mandarin, neroli, orange, patchouli, petitgrain, rose, rosewood and ylang ylang.

Tea or ti tree—
Melaleuca
alternifolia
(Myrtaceae family)

Tea tree is indigenous to Australia and has long been part of Aboriginal medicine. The oil was introduced to Europe in the early 1920s and used for its antiseptic qualities, particularly in the Second World War. The leaves and branches from which the oil is steam distilled have to be gathered by hand for the tree grows in snake-infested swampground and machine harvesting would be difficult. The yield from crops harvested in the Australian summer months from November to February is greater than that in the winter, but climatic conditions and the threat of bush fires may affect the crop. The massive worldwide increase in interest in the therapeutic properties of tea tree, especially amongst the medical profession, means that demand is overtaking supply and, although currently not an expensive essential oil, it is likely that the price will rise considerably in the not-too-distant future.

Chemical constituents   Alcohols and terpenes form the main constituents of tea tree oil. A large amount of the alcohol terpinen-4-ol with smaller amounts of α-terpineol and linalol, together with the monoterpenes, d-limonene, myrcene, phellandrene and pinene, and the sesquiterpenes, α-terpinene, γ-terpinene, sabinene and β-caryophyllene, combine to make the oil a powerful antiseptic, antibacterial, antiviral, antifungal and antimicrobial agent. Altman (1989) found that tea tree was 11 times more effective as a disinfectant and antiseptic than phenols, and Pena's early (1962) investigations showed its effectiveness in treating trichomonal and candidal infections of the vagina by means of tampons and douches. Likewise, Belaiche (1985a) demonstrated its action against *Candida albicans*, while Carson and Riley (1994) found that tea tree inhibited the actions not only of *C. albicans*, but also of *Escherichia coli, Staphylococcus aureus, Bacteroides fragilis, Mycobacterium smegmatis* and *Clostridium perfringens*. Belaiche (1985b) also used tea tree oil to treat skin infections such as staphylococcal acne, staphylococcal and streptococcal impetigo and *C. albicans*. Zarno (1994) recommends tea tree as the oil of first choice for candidiasis, and it can be administered in proprietary pessary form or on tampons soaked in tea tree solution for women with vaginal thrush. Suprapubic massage or compresses of tea tree may relieve cystitis, and the addition of a few drops to a suitable cream could alleviate the itching, inflammation and possible secondary infections associated with candidal napkin rash in the neonate.

Work is ongoing into the value of the oil as an immunostimulant, especially with people who are human immunodeficiency virus positive.

Sellar (1992, p. 159) suggests that preoperative and postoperative full-body massage with oil of tea tree may help to strengthen the body and reduce shock, as well as acting prophylactically against opportunistic infections; midwives could consider perioperative prophylactic baths for women booked for Caesarean section. Inhalations could also be given to women at risk of or showing signs of chest infection following anaesthetic.

Dangers Tea tree oil appears to be non-toxic and non-irritant. However, although it has been used successfully to treat skin disorders, it has also been reported to cause dermatitis in some individuals, particularly after prolonged application (De Groot and Weyland, 1993; Knight and Hausen, 1994). In Knight and Hausen's research the eczema and vesiculation that occurred in seven patients was most commonly found to be an allergy to *d*-limonene, with some allergy to α-terpinene and terpinen-4-ol.

Blends Tea tree oil has a strong medicinal aroma which blends well with cinnamon, cypress, eucalyptus, ginger, lavender, lemon, lemongrass, mandarin, marjoram, nutmeg, orange, rosemary, tangerine and thyme.

Ylang ylang—
Cananga odorata
(Anonaceae
family)
Ylang ylang essential oil is produced from the flowers of the tree, but there are several different grades obtained and only the purest should be used in therapeutic aromatherapy. It has a sweet floral and very heady aroma which can make some people feel nauseated.

Chemical constituents   Linalol (up to 30 per cent), geraniol and farnesol (alcohols) contribute towards the reputation of ylang ylang as an antidepressant and general tonic, while the ester benzyl acetate and the phenols eugenol and safrole aid its sedative action. The monoterpene pinene and the sesquiterpene cadinene, together with the phenols, assist in the antiseptic and antibacterial properties, which seem particularly effective with gastrointestinal infections. The alcohols and the cadinene are hypotensive.

Ylang ylang is renowned as a treatment for emotionally related conditions such as stress, panic, anxiety, sexual problems and hypertension. It appears to be safe to use in pregnancy in small doses and can help women who are very nervous and worried about their approaching labour.

Dangers   The high price of the superior grades of ylang ylang oil mean that it is open to adulteration with the inferior Cananga oil or other additions such as coconut oil. Ryman (1991, p. 218) suggests standing the bottle of oil in the refrigerator for, a short while for, if it is adulterated, it will thicken and become cloudy.

The aroma can be overpowering for some clients and it should be used in small doses intermittently; prolonged use may be stimulating rather than relaxing.

Blends   Ylang ylang blends well with lighter oils, which can subdue its intensity. These include bergamot, black pepper, camomile, grapefruit, jasmine, lavender, lemon, lime, marjoram, melissa, neroli, orange, patchouli, petitgrain, rose, rosewood and sandalwood.

Carrier or base oils

Essential oils are highly concentrated and, with only a very few exceptions, should rarely be used neat on the skin. This applies equally to using the oils in a massage blend or in the bath. The essential oils should be diluted into a good quality vegetable oil; mineral oils are not used as they do not allow the essential oil to absorb into the skin adequately, and may also contain lanolin to which some people are allergic.

The carrier oil serves as a lubricant when performing massage, enabling the hands of the practitioner to glide over the skin surface smoothly without friction. Different carrier oils are used for different purposes, but common to all is the need for the carrier to be 100 per cent pure and without an odour that could overpower the aromas of the essential oils.

Most carrier oils contain vitamins and minerals, and the texture will moisturize the skin. They may be produced from the nuts, seeds, beans or kernels of a variety of plants.

The following carrier oils are a few of the more commonly used oils, although there is a wide range of different ones from which to choose.

Almond, sweet—
Prunus amygdalis

Sweet almond oil is derived from the kernels of the almonds by warm pressing; it should not be confused with the bitter almond, the oil of which may contain prussic acid or cyanide (hydrocyanic acid) produced during the extraction process. Sweet almond trees have pink blossom, whereas bitter almond trees have white blossom. The oil is usually pale yellow, although the colour can vary according to the time of harvesting, from a greenish tinge to a deep gold. Completely colourless sweet almond oil is likely to have been refined and will no longer contain the vitamins A, B_1, B_2, B_6 and E, or the minerals and the monounsaturated and polyunsaturated fatty acids present in unrefined almond oil.

Sweet almond is one of the most popular carrier oils used in aromatherapy and is not overly expensive; the vitamin E content helps to preserve the oil. It is slightly sticky in texture and can be used on its own or mixed with another carrier oil. It will nourish the skin and is thought to be useful in cases of eczema and other irritations.

Apricot kernel—
Prunus armeniaca

Apricot oil is extracted from the seed kernels and is high in essential fatty acids, although, unlike the fruit, it does not contain many vitamins. The oil is light in texture, particularly suited to facial massage, and to dry, sensitive or mature skins as it is absorbed easily.

Avocado—
Persea americana

Mechanical pressing followed by centrifugal extraction is used to obtain avocado oil from the flesh of the fruit, grown largely in Mexico and in other parts of the southern United States and South America. The unrefined oil is a deep green colour and full of vitamins, lecithin, protein and essential fatty acids. It has a tendency to become cloudy and thick and, when cold, to solidify (although gentle warming of the bottle with the hands will reverse this process), leading producers in the cosmetics industry to refine the oil, which is then not suitable for use in aromatherapy.

The thick consistency and expensive price of avocado oil usually result in practitioners blending it with another carrier such as almond or grapeseed oil, but this does enhance the skin-nourishing properties of the final blend.

Avocado oil may be a pleasant addition to a blend to be used for abdominal massage in pregnancy, possibly helping to prevent striae gravidarum.

Grapeseed—
Vitis vinferi

This oil is obtained from the seeds of grapes, often imported from wine-growing areas in Europe. It is a yellow-green colour and very light in texture, without any noticeable odour. Grapeseed is universally used in aromatherapy for its non-greasy, silky feeling and because it is inexpensive, even more so than sweet almond oil. However, most grapeseed oils available on the market have been refined and lack the original nutrients, so it is wise to mix it with another, more nourishing, carrier for best effects.

Peach kernel—
Prunus persica

Peach kernel oil is similar to apricot kernel and is high in monounsaturates and polyunsaturates and vitamin E, making it good for facial massage. This is especially so as it is thought to stimulate secretion of the body's own naturally occurring oils and to encourage skin suppleness and elasticity; this could also be beneficial for abdominal massage in pregnancy.

Sesame seed—
Sesamum indicum

The oil is extracted from the seeds, which can yield up to 60 per cent pure oil. It is light and has virtually no odour, and has the advantage of washing out of towels better than grapeseed or sweet almond oil. As it is a mono-unsaturated oil it will retain its freshness longer than some other oils and will not go rancid in strong sunlight or excessive heat. Indeed, sesame oil can act as a fairly good sunfilter and is about 10 per cent more effective than many other carriers.

The oil can be used as a carrier on its own or mixed with another, and moisturizes dry skin.

Wheatgerm—
Triticum vulgare

Cold expression of the wheatgerm is performed to extract this dark orange-brown oil which is thick, rich and very nourishing, containing vitamin E and essential fatty acids. The vitamin E makes wheatgerm oil a natural antioxidant, i.e. it helps to prevent the deterioration that may occur when the oil is exposed to oxygen, light or temperature changes. Adding a small proportion (10–25 per cent) of wheatgerm to another base oil will enrich it, making it useful for dry skins or scar tissue and burns, and will prolong the 'shelf-life' of a carrier into which has been added essential oils.

There are many other carrier oils, but those outlined above are easily available, in the main relatively inexpensive and offer a versatile selection for the purposes of aromatherapy. Other base oils include borage, calendula, carrot, evening primrose, hazelnut, jojoba and macadamia nut oil.

Conclusion

Aromatherapy offers a wonderful range of fragrant essences which can be used to the benefit of the mother during pregnancy, labour and the puerperium, and for the baby. The therapy lends itself to incorporation into midwifery practice and, indeed, it is the belief and the wish of the author that it should become a part of normal midwifery practice. The use of massage, with or without essential oils, should be included in all programmes of initial preparation for midwives; in-depth modules that enable midwives to relate principles of aromatherapy to their practice should be offered as part of ongoing education, either as refresher courses or as units of study within post-registration diploma and degree programmes. Those midwives who are especially interested should be enabled to develop a specialist role as a midwife-aromatherapist so that they can act as a resource for other staff and offer a service to the mothers.

Midwives are working in an exciting time, when the implementation of 'Changing Childbirth' (Department of Health, 1993) encourages innovative practice to enhance the care of mothers and families. Aromatherapy can be utilized to offer additional strategies for physiological disorders, to relax women and to nurture them. We need to act as advocates for the women so that their memories of childbearing are as positive as possible. Aromatherapy is one way of working towards achieving that.

Appendix I: Essential Oils Suitable for Pregnancy and Childbirth

Essential oil	Uses in childbirth	Precautions
Basil	Pain relief in labour Chest infections, sinus congestion Retained placenta Postnatal 'blues'	Pregnancy Sensitive skin High doses
Benzoin	Cystitis Colic, flatulence, constipation Coughs, colds, sore throats Wound healing Stress, tension, anxiety	Sensitive skin
Bergamot	Cystitis, urinary tract infection Indigestion, colic, flatulence Viral infections Acne Pain relief in labour	Sunbathing
Black pepper	Pain relief in labour Bruising Constipation	Renal disease Women on diuretics Sensitive skin

Camomile	Cystitis, urinary tract infections Ophthalmia neonatorum Wound healing, sore nipples Pain relief in labour Backache, headache, afterpains Inducing rest and sleep	Pregnancy until term Sensitive skin
Clary sage	Respiratory infections Pain relief in labour Stress, depression	Pregnancy Care if driving Potentiates alcohol
Eucalyptus	Respiratory infections Cystitis	Sensitive skin Ingestion Epilepsy Hypertension With homoeopathy
Frankincense	Respiratory infections Urinary tract infections Anxiety in labour or postnatally	Pregnancy until term
Geranium	Oedema Pain relief in labour Sore nipples or perineum	Ensure purity
Ginger	Nausea and vomiting Diarrhoea, flatulence	Sensitive skin Sunlight
Grapefruit	Depression, stress, anxiety Nausea and vomiting, pica	Citrus allergy Store in refrigerator
Jasmine	Pain relief in labour Postnatal depression	Pregnancy Ensure purity
Juniper berry	Postnatal oedema	Pregnancy History of renal disease Hypertension
Lavender	Pain relief in labour Headache Poor uterine action Wound healing	Hypotension Epidural anaesthesia Pregnancy until term
Lemon	Infections Anaemia? Hypertension Gastric acidity	Sensitive skin
Lemongrass	Infections Pain relief in labour Inadequate lactation Heartburn, flatulence Loss of appetite	Sensitive skin

Lime	Depression, anxiety Loss of appetite, pica	Sunlight
Mandarin	Constipation Aids relaxation	Citrus allergy
Marjoram	Constipation, colic Pain relief in labour Colds, influenza	Pregnancy
Neroli	Stress, anxiety, depression Poor uterine action Reduced libido postnatally Insomnia	Care if driving
Nutmeg	Digestive complaints Pain relief in labour	*Never* in pregnancy
Orange	Hypertension Insomnia, stress Nausea and vomiting Constipation, colic Oedema	Citrus allergy
Patchouli	Poor libido Wound healing	Quality (?adulteration)
Petitgrain	Mood swings, stress Transition in labour Gastric discomfort	Skin sensitivity
Rose	Enhance contractions Depression, insomnia	Pregnancy
Rosemary	Stimulation, aids concentration Pain in labour Hypotension Hair care	Pregnancy Hypertension Epilepsy
Rosewood	Hypertension, pre-eclampsia Mood enhancer, relaxant	Purity
Sandalwood	Cystitis, urinary tract infections Genital infection Respiratory infections Poor libido	Purity Clinical depression
Tea tree	Vaginal infections Wound infections Respiratory infections	Skin irritation
Ylang ylang	Relaxation, stress Hypertension Antidepressant	Purity

Appendix II: Glossary of Terms and Properties of Essential Oils

Analgesic	pain relieving
Antacid	combats acidity
Antibiotic	combats bacterial infection
Anticoagulant	prevents blood clotting
Antidepressant	relieves depression
Antidontalgic	relieves toothache
Antiemetic	combats nausea and vomiting
Antimicrobial	fights microbial infection
Antiphlogistic	reduces inflammation
Antiseptic	controls infection
Antispasmodic	relieves cramp
Antisudorific	reduces sweating
Antiviral	fights viral infection
Aperitif	stimulates appetite
Aphrodisiac	increases sexual desire
Astringent	tightens and binds tissues
Balsamic	reduces and softens mucus
Bechic	eases coughing
Cardiac	stimulates heart
Carminative	encourages expulsion of flatus
Cephalic	stimulates, clears the mind
Cholagogue	increases bile secretion
Cicatrisant	helps formation of scar tissue
Cytoprophylactic	encourages growth of new cells
Decongestant	reduces mucus production
Deodorant	destroys odour
Depurative	purifies the blood
Digestive	aids digestion
Diuretic	stimulates micturition
Emmenagogue	induces uterine bleeding
Expectorant	clears excess mucus from bronchioles
Febrifuge	reduces pyrexia
Fungicide	fights fungal infections

Galactagogue	encourages lactation
Haemostatic	stops haemorrhage
Hepatic	stimulates liver and gallbladder
Hypertensive	increases blood pressure
Hypotensive	lowers blood pressure
Laxative	encourages bowel movements
Parturient	eases labour and delivery
Rubefacient	increases circulation, warming
Sedative	calming
Stimulant	increases energy and adrenaline
Stomachic	relieves gastric disorders
Sudorific	increases sweating
Uterine	tonic for the uterus
Vasoconstrictor	contracts blood vessel walls
Vasodilator	dilates blood vessel walls

Appendix III: Useful Addresses

Aromatherapy Organizations Council
3 Latymer Close
Braybrooke
Market Harborough
Leics
LE16 8LN
Tel: 01858 434242

'Umbrella' organization for most of the main aromatherapy bodies and schools

Aromatherapy World
Hinckley and District Hospital and Health Centre
The Annexe
Mount Road
Hinckley
Leics
LE10 1AG
Tel: 01455 637987

British Complementary Medicine Association
St Charles' Hospital
Exmoor Street
London W10 6DZ
Tel: 0181 964 1205

Holds registers of complementary therapy organizations

Institute for Complementary Medicine
PO Box 194
London SE16 1QZ
Tel: 0171 237 5165

Holds registers of individual practitioners of complementary medicine: good-sized library

International Journal of Aromatherapy
PO Box 746
Hove
East Sussex
BN3 2BD
Tel: 01273 772479

Natural Therapies Database UK
The Granary
Sladmore Farm
Cryers Hill Road
High Wycombe
Bucks
HP15 6LL

Publishes two quarterly volumes of research findings (aromatherapy and bodywork); will also conduct individual searches

Research Council for Complementary Medicine
60 Great Ormond Street
London WC1N 3JF
Tel: 0171 833 8897

Offers literature searches on complementary medicine. Access to many international databases

University of Greenwich, School of Health
Elizabeth Raybould Centre
Bow Arrow Lane
Dartford
Kent
DA2 6PJ
Tel: 0181 331 9169 (Registry)

Offers a Diploma of Higher Education in Complementary Therapy (Aromatherapy) for qualified health care professionals

References

Abdel Wahab S.M., Aboutel E.A., Wl-Zalabani S.M. *et al.* (1987) The essential oil of olibanum. *Planta Med* **3**: 382–384.

Abraham M., Devi N.S., & Sheela R. (1979) Inhibiting effect of jasmine flowers on lactation. *Indian J Med Res* **69**: 88–92.

Achterrath-Tuckermann U., Kunde R., Flaskamp E. *et al.* (1980) Pharmacological investigations with compounds of chamomile. Investigations on the spasmolytic effects of compounds of chamomile and Kamillosan on the isolated guinea pig ileum. *Planta Med* **39**: 38–50.

Adamson S. (1993) Hands-on therapy. *Health Visitor* **66**(2): 48–50.

Adamson-Macedo E.N. (1993) A small sample follow-up study of children who received tactile stimulation after pre-term birth: intelligence and achievements. *J Reprod Infant Psychol* **11**(3): 165–168.

Aertgeerts P., Abring M., Klaschka F. *et al.* (1985) Comparative testing of Kamillosan cream and steroidal (0.25% hydrocortisone, 0.75% fluocortin butyl ester) and non-steroidal (5% bufexamac) dermatologic agents maintenance therapy of eczematous diseases. *Z Hautkr* **60**(3): 270–277.

Agarwal I., Kharwal H.B. & Methela C.S. (1980) Chemical study and antimicrobial properties of essential oil of *Cymbopogon citratus* Linn. *Bull Med Ethnobot Res* **1**: 401–407.

Al-Hader A.A., Hasan Z.A. & Aqel M.B. (1994) Hyperglycaemic and insulin release inhibitory effects of *Rosmarinus officinalis*. *J Ethnopharmacol* **43**: 217–221.

Altman P.M. (1989) Australian tea tree oil—a natural antiseptic. *Aust J Biotech* **3**(4): 247–248.

Anonymous (1991) International News. *Int J Aromatherapy* **3**(4): 5.

Anonymous (1992) International News. *Int J Aromatherapy* **4**(3): 6.

Anonymous (1993a) International News. *Int J Aromatherapy* **5**(4): 2.

Anonymous (1993b) International News. *Int J Aromatherapy* **5**(2): 4–5.

Anonymous (1994a) International News. *Int J Aromatherapy* **6**(2): 2.

Anonymous (1994b) International News. *Int J Aromatherapy* **6**(3): 2.

Anonymous (1994c) *Aromatherapy Quarterly* No. 40: 13.

Aqel M.B. (1991) Relaxant effect of the

volatile oil of *Rosmarinus officinalis* on tracheal smooth muscle. *J Ethnopharmacol* **33**(1–2): 57–62.

Aqua Oleum (1993) *The Essential Oil Catalogue*. Aqua Oleum, Stroud.

Arcier M. (1992) *Aromatherapy*. Hamlyn, London.

Arkko P.J., Pakarinen A.J. & Kari-Koskinen O. (1983) Effects of whole body massage on serum protein, electrolyte and hormone concentrations, enzyme activities and haematological parameters. *Int J Sports Med* **4**: 265–267.

Asjes E. (1993) Managing epilepsy. *Int J Aromatherapy* **5**(3): 16–19.

Assaf M.H., Ali A.A., Makboul M.A. et al. (1987) Preliminary study of phenolic glycosides from *Origanum marjorana*: quantitative estimation of arbutin: cytotoxic activity of hydroquinone. *Planta Med* **53**(4): 343–345.

Badia P., Wesensten N., Lammers W. et al. (1990) Responsiveness to olfactory stimulation presented in sleep. *Physiol Behav* **48**(1): 87–90.

Balacs T. (1991a) Essential issues. *Int J Aromatherapy* **3**(4): 23–25.

Balacs T. (1991b) Research reports. *Int J Aromatherapy* **3**(4): 29–31.

Balacs T. (1992a) Safety in pregnancy. *Int J Aromatherapy* **4**(1): 12–15.

Balacs T. (1992b) Dermal crossing. *Int J Aromatherapy* **4**(2): 23–25.

Balacs T. (1992c) Well oiled pathways. *Int J Aromatherapy* **4**(3): 14–16.

Balacs T. (1993) Research reports. *Int J Aromatherapy* **5**(3): 34.

Barr J.S. & Taslitz N. (1970) The influence of back massage on autonomic functions. *Phys Ther* **50**(12): 1679–1691.

Barsoum G., Perry E.P. & Fraser I.A. (1990) Postoperative nausea is relieved by acupressure. *J R Soc Med* **83**: 86–89.

Bauer W.C. & Dracup K.A. (1987) Physiological effects of back massage in patients with acute myocardial infarction. *Focus Crit Care* **14**(6): 42–46.

Beal M.W. (1992) Acupuncture and related treatment modalities. Part 2: Applications to antepartal and intrapartal care. *J Nurse Midwifery* **37**(4): 260–268.

Belaiche P. (1985a) Treatment of vaginal infections of *Candida albicans* with the essential oil of *Melaleuca alternifolia* (Cheel). *Phytotherapy* **15**: 13–15.

Belaiche P. (1985b) Treatment of skin infections with the essential oil of *Melaleuca alternifolia* (Cheel). *Phytotherapy* **15**: 15–17.

Belluomini J., Litt R.C., Lee K.A. et al. (1994) Acupressure for nausea and vomiting of pregnancy: a randomized, blinded study. *Obstet Gynaecol* **84**(2): 245–248.

Bennett A., Stamford I.F., Tavares I.A. et al. (1988) The biological activity of eugenol, a major constituent of nutmeg (*Myristica fragrans*): studies on prostaglandins, the intestine and other tissues. *Phytother Res* **2**(3): 124–130.

Bensoussan A. (1991) *The Vital Meridian*. Churchill Livingstone, London.

Betts T. (1994) Sniffing the breeze. *Aromatherapy Quarterly* No. 40: 19–23.

Bilsland D. & Strong A. (1990) Allergic contact dermatitis from the essential oil of French marigold (*Tagetes patula*) in an aromatherapist. *Contact Dermatitis* **23**: 55–56.

Birch E.R. (1986) The experience of touch received during labour: postpartum perceptions of therapeutic value. *J Nurse Midwifery* **31**(6): 270–276.

Blackwell A.L. (1991) Anaerobic vaginosis. *Lancet* **337**(8736): 300 (letter).

Bowers-Clarke M. (1993) Baby massage. *New Generation* **12**(3): 4–5.

Boyd E.M. & Sheppard P. (1970) Nutmeg oil and camphene as inhaled expectorants. *Arch Otolaryngol* **92**(4): 372–378.

Boyland E. & Chasseau F. (1970) The effects of some carbonyl compounds on rat liver glutathione levels. *Biochem Pharmacol* **19**: 1526–1528.

Brandao F.M. (1986) Occupational allergy to lavender oil. *Contact Dermatitis* **15**(4): 249–250.

British Medical Association (1993) *Complementary Medicine: New Approaches to Good Practice*. Oxford University Press, Oxford.

Brud W. & Konopacka-Brud I. (1994) Rose oils. *Int J Aromatherapy* 6(2): 12–16.

Buchbauer G., Jirovetz L., Jager W. et al. (1991) Aromatherapy: evidence for sedative effects of the essential oil of lavender after inhalation. *Z Naturforsch C* 46(11–12): 1067–1072.

Buchbauer G., Jirovetz L., Jager W. et al. (1993) Fragrance compounds and essential oils with sedative effects upon inhalation. *J Pharm Sci* 82(6): 660–664.

Buckle J. (1993) Aromatherapy. Does it matter which lavender essential oil is used? *Nursing Times* 89(20): 32–35.

Budd S. (1992) Traditional Chinese medicine in obstetrics. *Midwives' Chronicle* 105(1253): 140–143.

Burns E. & Blamey C. (1994) Using aromatherapy in childbirth. *Nursing Times* 90(9): 54–60.

Calnan C.D. (1976) Cinnamon dermatitis from an ointment. *Contact Dermatitis* 2: 167–170.

Carola R., Harley J.P. & Noback C.R. (1992) *Human Anatomy and Physiology*, 2nd edn. McGraw Hill, New York.

Carson C.F. & Riley T.V. (1993) Antimicrobial activity of the essential oil of *Melaleuca alternifolia*. *Letters in Applied Microbiology* 16(2): 49–55.

Carson C.F. & Riley T.V. (1994) The antimicrobial activity of tea tree oil. *Med J Aust* 160: 236.

Classen C. & Howes D. (1993) Healing scents of the Andes. *Int J Aromatherapy* 5(4): 19–23.

Cripps R. (1994) How much do you touch? *Sainsburys Magazine* July: 47–50.

Cullen S.I., Tonkin A. & May F.E. (1974) Allergic contact dermatitis to compound tincture of benzoin spray. *J Trauma* 14(4): 348–350.

Dale A. & Cornwell S. (1994) The role of lavender oil in relieving perineal discomfort following childbirth: a blind randomized clinical trial. *J Adv Nurs* 19(1): 89–96.

Davis P. (1988) *Aromatherapy—An A–Z*. C.W. Daniel, Saffron Walden.

Day J.A., Mason R.R. & Chesrow S.E. (1987) Effect of massage on serum level of beta-endorphins and beta-lipotropin in healthy adults. *Phys Ther* 67(6): 926–930.

De Aloysio D. & Penacchioni P. (1992) Morning sickness control in early pregnancy by Neiguan point acupressure. *Obstet Gynaecol* 80(5): 852–854.

De Groot A.C. & Weyland J.W. (1993) Contact allergy to tea tree oil. *Contact Dermatitis* 28(2): 309.

De la Puerta R., Saenz M.T. & Garcia M.D. (1993) Choleretic effect of the essential oil from *Helichrysum picardii* Boiss. and reuter in rats. *Phytother Res* 7: 376–377.

Denholm J. (1992) Attitudes to Scent and Touch. *Aromatherapy World* Summer: 28.

Department of Health (1993) Changing Childbirth: Report of the Expert Maternity Group. HMSO, London.

Dooms-Goossens A., Degreef H., Holvoet C. & Maertens M. (1977) Turpentine-induced hypersensitivity to peppermint oil. *Contact Dermatitis* 3(6): 304–308.

Drury S. (1991) *Tea Tree Oil*. C.W. Daniel, Saffron Walden.

Dube S., Upadhyay P.D. & Tripathi S.C. (1989) Antifungal, physiochemical and insect-repelling activity of essential oil of *Ocimum basilicum*. *Can J Botany* 67(7): 2085–2087.

Dundee J.W. & Yang J. (1990) Prolongation of the antiemetic action of P6 acupuncture by acupressure in patients having cancer chemotherapy. *J R Soc Med* 83: 360–362.

Dundee J.W., Sourial F.B.R. & Ghaly R.G. (1988) P6 acupuncture reduces morning sickness. *J R Soc Med* 81(8): 456–457.

Elder T.D. et al. (1960) *Science* 132: 225–226.

Elisha N. *et al.* (1988) Effects of *Jasminum officinale* flowers on the central nervous system of the mouse. *Int J Crude Drug Res* **26**(4): 221–227.

Elson C.E., Underbakke G.L., Hanson P. *et al.* (1989) Impact of lemongrass oil, an essential oil, on serum cholesterol. *Lipids* **24**(8): 677–679.

Emeny P. (1994) Case study—diabetic gangrene. *Int J Aroma* **6**(1): 21.

Ernst E., Matrai A., Magyarosy L. *et al.* (1987) Massage causes changes in blood fluidity. *Physiotherapy* **73**(1): 43–45.

Evans A.T., Samuels S.N., Marshall C. *et al.* (1993) Suppression of pregnancy-induced nausea and vomiting with sensory afferent stimulation. *J Reprod Med* **38**(8): 603–606.

Falk-Filipsson A. (1993) *d*-Limonene exposure to humans by inhalation: uptake, distribution, elimination and effects on the pulmonary system. *J Toxicol Environ Health* **38**: 77–88.

Fang H.J., Su X.L., Liu H.Y. *et al.* (1989) Studies on the chemical components and anti-tumour action of the volatile oils from *Pelargonium graveolens*. *Yao Hsueh Hsueh Pao* **24**(5): 366–371.

Farrell M. (1994a) Jottings from journals. *Aromatherapy World* Summer 1994, p. 26.

Farrell M. (1994b) Phytomedicines—research and therapy with phytomedicines. European Scientific Cooperative on Phytotherapy. Third International Symposium. *Aromatherapy Quarterly* Summer 1994, pp. 29–32.

Farrow J. (1990) Massage therapy and nursing care. *Nursing Standard* **4**(17): 26–28.

Ferrell-Torry A.T. & Glick O.J. (1993) The use of therapeutic massage as a nursing intervention to modify anxiety and the perception of cancer pain. *Cancer Nurs* **16**(2): 93–101.

Field T.M., Schanburg S.M., Scadafi F. *et al.* (1986) Tactile/kinesthetic stimulation effects on preterm neonates. *Pediatrics* **77**(5): 654–658.

Field T., Morrow C., Vaideon C. *et al.* (1993) Massage reduces anxiety in child and adolescent psychiatric patients. *Int J Alternative Complementary Med* **11**(7): 22–27.

Fraser J. & Kerr J.R. (1993) Psychophysiological effects of back massage on elderly institutionalised patients. *J Adv Nurs* **18**: 238–245.

Gabbrielli G., Loggini F., Cioni P.L. *et al.* (1988) Activity of lavandino essential oil against non-tubercular opportunistic rapid growth mycobacteria. *Pharmacol Res Commun* December (supplement 5): 37–40.

Gamez M.J., Jimenez J., Navarro C. & Zarzuelo A. (1990) Study of the essential oil of *Lavandula dentata*. *Pharmazie* **45**: 69.

Garland D. (1995) The uses of hydrotherapy in today's midwifery practice. In *Complementary Therapies for Pregnancy and Childbirth* (D. Tiran & S. Mack, eds), pp. 113–126. Baillière Tindall, London.

Ginsberg F. & Famaey J.P. (1987) A double-blind study of topical massage with Rado-salil ointment in mechanical low-back pain. *J Int Med Res* **15**: 148–153.

Glowania H.J., Raulin C. & Soboda M. (1987) Effect of chamomile on wound healing—a clinical double-blind study. *Z Hautkr* **62**(17): 1267–1271.

Goldberg J., Sullivan S.J. & Seaborne D.E. (1992) The effect of two intensities of massage on H-reflex amplitude. *Phy Ther* **72**(6): 449–457.

Guerra P., Aguilar A., Urbina F. *et al.* (1987) Contact dermatitis to geraniol in a leg ulcer. *Contact Dermatitis* **16**(5): 298–299.

Guillemain J., Rousseau A. & Delaveau P. (1989) Neurodepressive effects of the essential oil of *Lavandula angustifolia* Mill. *Ann Pharm Fr* **47**(6): 337–343.

Gundidza M., Chinyanganya F. & Mavi S. (1993) Antimicrobial activity of the essential oil from *Eucalyptus maidenii*. *Planta Med* **59** (supplement): A705.

Gurr F.W. & Scroggie J.G. (1965) Eucalyptus oil poisoning treated by dialysis and mannitol infusion, with an appendix on the analysis of biological fluids for alcohol and eucalyptol. *Australas Ann Med* **14**(3): 238–249.

Hajji F. & Fkih-Tetouani S. (1993) Antimicrobial activity of twenty one eucalyptus essential oils. *Fitoterapia* **64**(1): 71–77.

Harding J. (1994a) In profile: Dr Steve Van Toller. *Int J Aromatherapy* **6**(1): 4–7.

Harding J. (1994b) The scent trail. *Int J Aromatherapy* **6**(3): 8–11.

Hardy M. (1991) Sweet scented dreams. *Int J Aromatherapy* **3**(2): 12–13.

Hartnoll G., Moore D. & Douek D. (1993) Near fatal ingestion of oil of cloves. *Arch Dis Child* **69**: 392–393.

Hedstrom L.W. & Newton N. (1986) Touch in labour: a comparison of cultures and eras. *Birth* **13**(3): 181–186.

Henry J., Rusius C.W., Davies M. & Veazey-French T. (1994) Lavender for night sedation of people with dementia. *Int J Aromatherapy* **6**(2): 28–30.

Hethelyi E., Kaposi P., Domonkos J. & Kernoczi Z. (1987) GC/MS investigation of the essential oil of *Rosmarinus officinalis* L. *Acta Pharm Hung* **57**(3–4): 159–169.

Hill C.F. (1993) Is massage beneficial to critically ill patients in intensive care? A critical review. *J Intens Crit Care Nurs* **9**: 116–121.

Hirsch A. (1992a) The good old smells. *Int J Aromatherapy* **4**(3): 7–9.

Hirsch A. (1992b) Scentsation. *Int J Aromatherapy* **4**(1): 16–17.

Hmamouch M., Tantaoui-Elaraki A., Es-Safu N. & Agoumi A. (1990) Illustration of antibacterial and antifungal properties of Eucalyptus essential oils. *Plantes Med Phytotherapie* **24**(4): 278–289.

Holmes P. (1994) Rose—the water goddess. *Int J Aromatherapy* **6**(2): 8–11.

Hovind H. & Nielson S.L. (1974) Effect of massage on blood flow in skeletal muscle. *Scand J Rehabil Med* **6**: 74–77.

Hyde E. (1989) Acupressure therapy for morning sickness. A controlled clinical trial. *J Nurse Midwifery* **34**(4): 171–178.

Imberger I., Rupp J., Karamat C. & Buchbauer G. (1993) Effects of essential oils on human attentional processes. *Programme Abstracts—24th International Symposium on Essential Oils.*

International School of Aromatherapy (1993) *A Safety Guide on the Use of Essential Oils.* Natural by Nature, London.

Isherwood D. (1994) Baby massage groups. *New Generation* **12**(3): 4–6.

Jager W., Buchbauer G. & Jirovetz L. (1992) Evidence of the sedative effects of neroli oil, citronellal and phenylethyl acetate on mice. *J Essent Oil Res* **4**: 387–394.

James W.D., White S.W. & Yanklowitz B. (1984) Allergic contact dermatitis to compound tincture of benzoin. *J Am Acad Dermatol* **5**(1): 847–850.

Janssens J., Laekeman G.M., Pieters L.A. et al. (1990) Nutmeg oil: identification and quantitation of its most active constituents as inhibitors of platelet aggregation. *J Ethnopharmacol* **29**(2): 179–188.

Jenson O.K. Nielson F.F. & Vosmar L. (1990) An open study comparing manual therapy with the use of cold packs in the treatment of post-traumatic headache. *Cephalagia* **10**: 241–249.

Jirovetz L., Buchbauer G., Jager W. et al. (1992) Analysis of fragrance compounds in blood samples of mice by gas chromatography, mass spectrometry, GC/FTIR and GC/AES after inhalation of sandalwood oil. *Biomed Chromatogr* **6**(3): 133–134.

Johanson R.B., Spencer S.A., Rolfe P. et al. (1992) Effect of post-delivery care on neonatal body temperature. *Acta Paediatr* **81**(11): 859–863.

Johnson E. (1995) Shiatsu. In *Complementary Therapies for Pregnancy and Childbirth* (D. Tiran & S. Mack, eds). Baillière Tindall, London. pp. 127–152.

Jori A., Bianchietti A. & Prestini P.E. (1969) Effects of essential oils on drug metabolism. *Biochem Pharmacol* **18**(9): 2081–2085.

Joshi D.J., Dikshit R.K. & Mansuri S.M. (1987) Gastrointestinal actions of garlic oil. *Phytother Res* **1**(3): 140–141.

Kaada B. & Torsteinbo O. (1989) Increase of plasma beta-endorphins in connective tissue massage. *Gen Pharmacol* **20**(4): 487–489.

Kallan C. (1991) Probing the power of common scents. *Prevention* **43**(10): 38.

Karamat E., Imberger J., Buchbauer G. *et al.* (1992) Excitory and sedative effects of essential oils on human reaction time performance. *Chem Senses* **17**(4): 847.

Kikuchi A., Tsuchiya T., Tanida M. *et al.* (1989) Stimulant-like ingredients in absolute jasmine. *Chem Senses* **14**(2): 304.

Kirk-Smith, M. & Stretch, D. (1994) Clinical trials in aromatherapy. *Int J Aromatherapy* **6**(1): 32–35.

Kirwin B. (1993) Case study: oral candidiasis. *Int J Aroma* **5**(4): 24.

Knasko S.C. (1992) Ambient odor's effect on creativity, mood and perceived health. *Chem Senses* **17**(1): 27–35.

Knight T.E. & Hausen B.M. (1994) Melaleuca oil (tea tree) dermatitis. *J Am Acad Dermatol* **30**(3): 423–427.

Kobal G. *et al.* (1992) Differences in human chemosensory evoked potentials to olfactory and somatosensory chemical stimuli presented to left and right nostrils. *Chemical Senses* **17**(3): 233–244.

Kovar K.A., Gropper B., Friess D. & Svendsen A. (1987) Blood levels of 1.8 cineole and locomotor activity of mice after inhalation and oral administration of rosemary oil. *Planta Med* **53**(4): 315–318.

Kubler S. & Wabner D. (1994) A museum for the rose. *Aromatherapy Quarterly* **41**: 21–25.

Kuhn C.M., Schanberg S.M., Field T. *et al.* (1991) Tactile–kinesthetic stimulation effects on sympathetic and adreno-cortical function in preterm infants. *J Pediatr* **119**(3): 434–440.

Lavabre M. (1990) *Aromatherapy Workbook.* Healing Arts Press, Rochester, USA.

Lawless J. (1992) *The Encyclopaedia of Essential Oils.* Element Books, Shaftesbury.

Lawless J. (1994) Scent, soul and psyche. *Aromatherapy Quarterly* No. 42, pp. 17–21.

Le May A. (1986) The human connection. *Nursing Times* 19 November 1986: 28–30.

Lesesne C.B. (1992) The postoperative use of wound adhesives. Gum mastic *versus* benzoin, USP. *J Dermatol Surg Oncol* **18**(11): 990.

Lewis L. (1995) Caring for the carers. *Modern Midwife* **5**(2): 7–10.

Lichy R. & Herzberg E. (1993) *The Waterbirth Handbook.* Gateway Books, Bath.

Lorenzetti B.B., Souza G.E., Sarti S.J. *et al.* (1991) Myrcene mimics the peripheral analgesic activity of lemongrass tea. *J Ethnopharmacol* **34**(1): 43–48.

Lorig T.S. *et al.* (1993) Visual event-related potentials during odour labelling. *Chemical Senses* **18**(4): 379–387.

Lyrenas S., Lutsch H., Hetta J. *et al.* (1987) Acupuncture before delivery: effect on labor. *Gynecol Obstet Invest* **24**(4): 217–224.

McArdle M. (1992) Rosewood in pre-eclampsia. *Int J Aromatherapy* **4**(1): 33 (letter).

McGeorge B.C. & Steele M.C. (1991) Allergic contact dermatitis of the nipple from Roman chamomile ointment. *Contact Dermatitis* **24**(2): 139–140.

McGilvery C. & Reed J. (1993) *Essential Aromatherapy.* Acropolis Books, Leicester.

Mack, S. (1995) Attitudes to complementary therapy. In Tiran, D. and Mack, S. (eds) *Complementary Therapies for Pregnancy and Childbirth*, pp. 265–282. Baillière Tindall, London.

McKechnie A.A., Wilson F., Watson N.

& Scott D. (1983) Anxiety states: a preliminary report on the value of connective tissue massage. *J Psychosom Res* **27**(2): 125–129.

Maclean M. (1993) Classroom harmony. *Int J Aromatherapy* **5**(2): 10–11.

Manley C.H. (1993) Psychophysiological effect of odour. *Crit Rev Food Sci Nutr.* **33**(1): 57–62.

Mann R.J. (1982) Benzoin sensitivity. *Contact Dermatitis* **8**(4): 263.

Marsden K. (1991) The aromatherapy phenomenon. *Int J Aroma* **3**(4): 6–9.

Mayo W.L. (1992) Australian tea tree oil: a summary of medical, pharmacological and alternative health research and writings. *J Alternative Complementary Med* **10**(12): 13–16.

Meyer J. (1970) Accidents due to tanning cosmetics with a base of bergamot oil. *Bull Soc Fr Dermatol Syphiligr* **77**(6): 881–884.

Minchin M. (1994) Geranium. When there were no more cabbage leaves. *Australian Lactation Consultants Association (ALCA) News* **5**(1): 8–10.

Misra N., Batra S. & Mishra D. (1988) Fungitoxic properties of the essential oil of *Citrus lemon* (L.) Burm. against a few dermatophytes. *Mycoses* **31**(7): 380–382.

Miyake Y., Nakagawa M. & Asakura Y. (1991) Effect of odours on humans (1). Effects on sleep latency. *Chem Senses* **16**(1): 183.

Miyazaki Y., Takeuchi S., Yatagi M. & Kobayashi S. (1991) The effect of essential oils on mood in humans. *Chem Senses* **16**(1): 184.

Montagu A. (1986) *Touching: the Human Significance & Skin*, 3rd edn., London, Harper and Row.

Morelli M., Seaborne D.E. & Sullivan S.J. (1990) Changes in H-reflex amplitude during massage of triceps surae in healthy subjects. *Orthop Sports Phy Ther* **12**(2): 55–59.

Mumm A.H., Morens D.M. & Diwan A.R. (1993) Zoster after shiatsu massage. *Lancet* **341**: 447.

Naganuma M., Hirose S., Nakayama Y.

et al. (1985) A study of the phototoxicity of lemon oil. *Arch Dermatol Res* **278**(1): 31–36.

Nasel C., Nasel B., Samec P. *et al.* (1994) Functional imaging of effects of fragrances on the human brain after prolonged inhalation. *Chem Senses* **19**(4): 359–364.

National Association of Health Authorities and Trusts (1993) *Complementary Therapies in the NHS.* NAHAT, London.

Neilan A. (1994) Case study: oral thrush. *Int J Aroma* **6**(2): 24.

Nissen H.P., Biltz H. & Kreysel H.W. (1988) Profilometry, a method for the assessment of the therapeutic effectiveness of Kamillosan ointment. *Z Hautkr* **63**(3): 184–190.

North L. (1994) Letters. *Aromatherapy World* Autumn: 11.

Ogunlana E.O., Hoglund S., Onawunmi G. & Skold O. (1987) Effects of lemongrass oil on the morphological characteristics and peptidoglycan synthesis of *Escherichia coli* cells. *Microbios* **50**: 43–59.

Olsen P. & Thorup I. (1984) Neurotoxicity in rats dosed with peppermint oil and pulegone. *Arch. Toxical. Suppl.* **7**: 408–409.

Onawunmi G.O. (1988) *In vitro* studies on the antibacterial activity of phenoxyethanol in combination with lemongrass oil. *Pharmazie* **43**(1): 42–43.

Onawunmi G.O. (1989) Antifungal activity of lemongrass oil. *Int J Crude Drug Res* **27**(2): 121–126.

Onawunmi G.O. & Ogunlana E.O. (1986) A study of the antibacterial activity of the essential oil of lemon grass (*Cymbopogon citratus*) (D.C.) Stapf. *Int J Crude Drug Res* **24**(2): 64–68.

Onawunmi G.O., Yisak W.A. & Ogunlana E.O. (1984) Antibacterial constituents in the essential oil of *Cymbopogon citratus* (D.C.) Stapf. *Ethnopharmacology* **12**(3): 279–286.

Orafidiya L.O. (1993) The effect of auto-oxidation of lemongrass oil on its antibacterial activity. *Phytother Res* **7**: 269–271.

Page C. (1994) Stretching the frontiers of health. *Aromatherapy Quarterly* No. 43: pp. 19–21.

Pages N., Fournier G., Le Luyer F. & Marques M.C. (1990) Essential oils and their potential teratogenic properties: the case of *Eucalyptus globulus* essential oil—preliminary study on mice. *Plantes Med Phytother* **24**(1): 21–26.

Parys B.T. (1983) Chemical burns resulting from contact with peppermint oil mar: a case report. *Burns, Including Thermal Injury* **9**(5): 374–375.

Patel S. & Wiggins J. (1980) Eucalyptus oil poisoning. *Arch Dis Child* **55**(5): 405–406.

Pena E.F. (1962) *Melaleuca alternifolia* oil. Its use for trichomonas vaginitis and other vaginal infections. *Obstet Gynecol* **19**(6): 793–795.

Penoel D. (1992) *Eucalyptus smithii* essential oil and its uses in aromatic medicine. *Br J Phytother* **2**(4): 154–159.

Penoel D. (1994) Art and science. The aromatic triptych revisited. *Int J Aromatherapy* **6**(3): 5–7.

Perez Raya M.D., Utrilla M.P., Navarro M.C. & Jimenez J. (1990) CNS activity of *Mentha rotundifolia* and *Mentha longifolia* essential oil in mice and rats. *Phytother Res* **4**(6): 232–234.

Price H., Lewith G. & Williams C. (1991) Acupressure as an anti-emetic in cancer chemotherapy. *Complementary Medicine Research* **5**(2): 93–94.

Price, S. (1992) The position of aromatherapy in European countries other than Britain. *Aromatherapy World* Summer 1992: pp. 16–17.

Price S. (1993) *The Aromatherapy Workbook*. Thorsons, Wellingborough.

Puustjarvi K., Airaksinen O. & Pontinen P.J. (1990) The effects of massage in patients with chronic tension headache. *Acupuncture and Electrotherapy Research* **15**: 159–162.

Rademaker M. & Kirby J.D.T. (1987)

Contact dermatitis to a skin adhesive. *Contact Dermatitis* **16**(5): 297–298.

Rangelov A., Pisanetz M., Toreva D. & Kosev R. (1988) Experimental study of the cholagogic and choleretic action of some of the basic ingredients of essential oils on laboratory animals. *Folia Med (Plovdiv)* **30**(4): 30–38.

Renn B. (1994) Environmental fragrancing. *Aromatherapy World* Spring 1994: p. 25.

Roach B. (1985) Ginger root (*Zingibar officinale*). *California Association of Midwives Newsletter* **1**: 2.

Roberts A. & Williams J.M.G. (1992) The effect of olfactory stimulation on fluency, vividness of imagery and associated mood: a preliminary study. *Br J Med Psychol* **65**(2): 197–199.

Rothe A., Heine A. & Rebohle E. (1973) Oil from juniper berries as an occupational allergen for the skin and respiratory tract. *Berufsdermatosen* **21**(1): 11–16.

Rudski E., Grzywa Z. & Bruo W.S. (1976) Sensitivity to 35 essential oils. *Contact Dermatitis* **2**: 196–200.

Ryman D. (1991) *Aromatherapy—The Encyclopaedia of Plants and Oils and How They Help You*. Piatkus, London.

Safayhi H., Sabieraj J., Sailer E.R. & Ammon H.P.T. (1994) Chamazulene: an antioxidant-type inhibitor of leucotriene B_4 formation. *Planta Med* **60**: 410–413.

Schafer D. & Schafer W. (1981) Pharmacological studies with an ointment containing menthol, camphene and essential oils for broncholytic and secretolytic effects. *Arzneimittelforschung* **31**(1): 82–86.

Scott C. (1993) In Profile—Dr Jean Valnet. *Int J Aromatherapy* **5**(4): 10–13.

Sellar W. (1992) *The Directory of Essential Oils*. C.W. Daniel, Saffron Walden.

Seth G., Kokate C.K. & Varma K.C. (1976) Effect of essential oil of *Cymbopogon citratus* stapf. on the central nervous system. *Indian J Exp Biol* **14**(3): 370–371.

Sharma R., Bajaj A.K. & Singh K.G. (1987) Sandalwood dermatitis. *Int J Dermatol* **26**(9): 597.

Shemesh A.U. & Mayo W.L. (1991) Tea tree oil—natural antiseptic and fungicide. *J Alternative Complementary Med* **9**(12): 11–12.

Shrivastav P., Goerge K., Balasubramaniam N. *et al.* (1988) Suppression of puerperal lactation using jasmine flowers (*Jasminum sambac.*). *Aust N Z J Obstet Gynaecol* **28**(1): 68–71.

Sims S. (1986) Slow stroke back massage for cancer patients. *Nursing Times* **82**(13): 47–50.

Soliman F.M.., El-Kashoury E.A., Fathy M.M. & Gonaid M.H. (1994) Analysis and biological activity of the essential oil of *Rosmarinus officinalis* L. from Egypt. *Flavour Fragrance J* **9**: 29–33.

Somerville K.W., Richmond C.R. & Bell G.D. (1984) Delayed release peppermint oil capsules (Colpermin) for the spastic colon syndrome: a pharmokinetic study. *Br J Clin Pharmacol* **18**(4): 638–640.

Spoerke D.G., Vandenburg S.A., Smolinske S.C. *et al.* (1989) Eucalyptus oils; 14 cases of exposure. *Vet Hum Toxicol* **31**(2): 166–168.

Stannard D. (1989) Pressure prevents nausea. *Nursing Times* **85**(4): 33–34.

Steele J. (1992) Environmental fragrancing. *Int J Aromatherapy* **4**(2): 9–11.

Stephen J. (1994) Notes from a perfume workshop. *Aromatherapy Quarterly* No. 42: pp. 29–32.

Stevenson C. (1992) Orange blossom evaluation. *Int J Aromatherapy* **4**(3): 22–24.

Sugano H. (1989) Effects of odours on mental function. *Chem Senses* **14**(2): 303.

Sugano H. & Sato N. (1991) Psychophysiological studies of fragrance. *Chem Senses* **16**(1): 183–184.

Sullivan S.J., Williams L.R., Seaborne D.E. & Morelli M. (1991) Effects of massage on motorneuron excitability. *Phys Ther* **71**(8): 555–560.

Svoboda S.G. & Deans K.P. (1990) A study of the variability of rosemary and sage and their volatile oils on the British market: their antioxidant properties. *Flavour Fragrance J* **7**: 81–87.

Taddei I., Giachetti D., Taddei E. & Mantovani P. (1988) Spasmolytic activity of peppermint, sage and rosemary essences and their major constituents. *Fitoterapia* **59**(6): 463–468.

Tasev T., Toleva P. & Balabanova V. (1969) The neuro-psychic effect of Bulgarian rose, lavender and geranium. *Folia Med* **11**(5): 307–317.

Temple W.A., Smith N.A. & Beasley M. (1991) Management of oil of citronella poisoning. *J Clin Toxicol* **29**(2): 257–262.

Tiran D. & Mack S. (eds) (1995) *Complementary Therapies for Pregnancy and Childbirth.* Baillière Tindall, London.

Tisserand R. (1992) *The Art of Aromatherapy,* 2nd edn. C.W. Daniel, Saffron Walden.

Tisserand R. (1993) Aromatherapy today—part I. *Int J Aromatherapy* **5**(3): 26–29.

Tisserand R. & Balacs T. (1995) *Essential Oil Safety. A Guide for Health Professionals.* Churchill Livingstone, London.

Toaff M.E., Abramovici A., Sporn J. & Liban E. (1979) Selective oocyte degeneration and impaired fertility in rats treated with the aliphatic monoterpene Citral. *J Reprod Fertil* **55**: 347–352.

Tripathi R.C., Fekrat-Polacik B., Tripathi B.J. & Ernest J.T. (1990) An unusual necrotising dermatitis after a single application of topical benzoin and pressure bandage for enucleation of an eye. *Lens Eye Toxic Res* **7**(2): 173–178.

Tubaro A., Zilli C., Redaelli C. & Delia Loggia R. (1984) Evaluation of anti-inflammatory activity of a chamomile extract topical application. *Planta Med* **50**(4): 359.

UK Central Council (1992a) *The Scope of Professional Practice.* UK Central Council, London.

UK Central Council (1992b) *Standards*

for the Administration of Medicines. UK Central Council, London.

UK Central Council (1992c) *Code of Conduct for Nurses, Midwives and Health Visitors.* UK Central Council, London.

UK Central Council (1994) *A Midwife's Code of Practice.* UK Central Council, London.

Valnet J. (1982) *The Practice of Aromatherapy.* C.W. Daniel, Saffron Walden.

Van Ketel W.G. (1987) Allergy to *Matricaria chamomilla. Contact Dermatitis* **8**(2): 143.

Varendi H., Porter R.H. & Winberg J. (1994) *The Lancet* **344**(8928): 989–990.

Waymouth S. (1992) Case study—Essential hypertension. *Int J Aromatherapy* **4**(3): 29.

Wells R. & Tschudin V. (1994) *Wells' Supportive Therapies in Health Care.* Baillière Tindall, London.

Weyers W. & Brodbeck R. (1989) Skin absorption of volatile oils. Pharmokinetics. *Pharm Unserer Zeit* **18**(3): 82–86.

White-Traut R.C. & Nelson M.N. (1988) Maternally administered tactile, auditory, visual and vestibular stimulation: relationship to later interactions between mothers and premature infants. *Res Nurs Health* **11**: 31–39.

Woeber K. & Krombach M. (1969) Sensitisation from volatile oils (preliminary report). *Berufsdermatosen* **17**(6): 320–326.

Wong M. (1994) The healing touch. *Aromatherapy Quarterly* No. 42: pp. 13–15.

Worwood V. (1990) *The Fragrant Pharmacy.* Bantam Books, London.

Zakarya D., Fkih-Tetouani S. & Hajji F. (1993) Chemical composition—antimicrobial activity relationships of eucalyptus essential oils. *Plantes Med Phytother* **26**(4): 319–331.

Zarno V. (1994) Candidiasis. *Int J Aromatherapy* **6**(2): 20–23.

Zheng G., Kenney P. & Lam K.T. (1993) Potential anticarcinogenic natural products isolated from lemongrass oil and galanga root oil. *J Agric Food Chem* **41**(2): 153–156.

Further reading

Ashby N. (1994) Subtle anatomy and physiology. *Aromatherapy Quarterly* No. 40: pp. 29–31.

Mojay G. (1993) The Chinese Energetic Model. *Int J Aromatherapy* **5**(3): 9–12.

Sun D. (1994) The aroma of colour. *Aromatherapy World* Spring 1994: pp. 21–24.

Sweet B. & Tiran D. (1996) *Mayes' Midwifery*, 12th edn. Baillière Tindall, London.

Trevelyan J. & Booth B. (1995) *Complementary Medicine for Nurses, Midwives and Health Visitors.* MacMillan Press, London.

Wong M. (1994) Do plants have souls? Exploring the esoteric properties of essential oils. *Aromatherapy Quarterly* No. 41: pp. 33–35.

Index

Numbers in *italics* refer to illustrations or tables. Numbers in **bold** refer to main reference.